Unlock the Secrets of a Good Night's Rest

"This book is about self-healing. It teaches you to use your own physical movements and breath to overcome insomnia and get all the natural, restful sleep you need. In the process, you will heal your relationship with sleep. That means that your feelings about sleep and your attitudes toward sleep will change. Instead of dreading bedtime as a time of irritation, uncertainty, or disappointment, you will look forward to it as a time of comfort, pleasure, and peace." —From *The Insomnia Solution*

Praise for *The Insomnia Solution* and Michael Krugman's Sounder Sleep System™

"Engaging . . . accessible . . . very helpful . . . if you're having a problem sleeping, this may be your answer."
—Jim Stephens, PhD, PT, CFP, assistant professor, Physical Therapy Department, College of Health Professions, Temple University

"Great results." —*Fortune*

"Tiny, relaxing movements and dreamy rest. You'll feel smarter and you'll sleep better." —*Village Voice*

THE
INSOMNIA
SOLUTION

* * * * * * * * * * *

The Natural,
Drug-Free Way to a
Good Night's Sleep

Michael Krugman, MA, GCFP

WARNER BOOKS

NEW YORK · BOSTON

The program herein is not intended to replace the services of trained health professionals, or be a substitute for medical advice. You are advised to consult with your health care professional with regard to matters relating to your health, and in particular regarding matters that may require diagnosis or medical attention.

The excerpt on pages 292 and 293 is from "The Potent Self: A Study of Spontaneity and Compulsion" by Moshe Feldenkrais, published by Frog Lt. and Somatic Resources, copyright © 2002 by Michel Silice. Reprinted by permission of the publishers.

Sounder™, Sounder Sleep™, Sounder Sleep System™, Sominars™, and Mini-Moves™ are trademarks of Michael Krugman. Feldenkrais®, Feldenkrais Method®, Awareness Through Movement®, Functional Integration®, and Guild Certified Feldenkrais Teacher® are service marks of the Feldenkrais Guild® of North America.

Warner Books

Time Warner Book Group
1271 Avenue of the Americas, New York, NY 10020
Visit our Web site at www.twbookmark.com.

Printed in the United States of America

First Edition: August 2005
10 9 8 7 6 5 4 3 2 1

Library of Congress Cataloging-in-Publication Data
Krugman, Michael.
    The insomnia solution : the natural, drug-free way to a good night's sleep /
Michael Krugman. — 1st ed.
        p.   cm.
    ISBN 0-446-69324-3
    1. Insomnia—Popular works.   2. Sleep.   I. Title.
    RC548.K78 2005
    616.8'498206—dc22   2005000388

For Karen

Acknowledgments

★ ★ ★ ★

Thanks to my many colleagues and friends for their indispensable help, support, and inspiration during the gestation and writing of this book. Special thanks to Hiltrud Müller-Fehn for translation, Laura Scheufele for research assistance, Nyei Murez and Robbie Ofir for editorial support, Alex Candelaria Sedillos for photography, and High Desert Yoga, Albuquerque, and Karen Ann Swift for modeling. Thanks to Avri Glick, Dilys Garcia, Aliza Stewart, Peter Hasson, Jean Ashby, Charlotte Palumbo, Ginger Carney, Carol Meade, Christel Schulte, Patricio Simon, Janine Holenstein, Nora Karner, Ulfried Blaschek, Felicia Noëlle Trujillo, Marta Ballen, Garet Newell, Tina and Katarina Tribe, Claire Nettle, and many others for giving me the opportunity to share the gift. Last but not least, thanks to all those who have attended my classes, seminars, and retreats. You are my greatest inspiration.

Contents

★ ★★★ ★

Dear to us ever is the banquet, and the harp, and the dance, and changes of raiment, and the warm bath, and love, and sleep.

—*The Odyssey,* Book VIII

THE
INSOMNIA
SOLUTION

Introduction

★ ★ ★ ★ ★

Why America Can't Sleep

Enjoy the honey-heavy dew of slumber:
Thou hast no figures nor no fantasies,
Which busy care draws in the brains of men;
Therefore thou sleep'st so sound.
            —SHAKESPEARE, *Julius Caesar*

Do you have trouble sleeping? If so, you are not alone. In a recent poll conducted by the National Sleep Foundation, more than half the respondents had symptoms of insomnia at least a few nights a week. Thirty-five percent said that they experienced symptoms every night or almost every night in the past year. Since September 11, 2001, sales of sleeping pills have soared by 25 percent, and anti-anxiety drugs are up nearly 10 percent according to the chief of integrative medicine at Memorial Sloan-Kettering Cancer Center in New York. And Dr. Carl E. Hunt, director of the National Center on Sleep Disorders Research, estimates that there are as many as seventy million problem sleepers in the United States. By all accounts, the United States is suffering from an epidemic of sleeplessness.

We may chuckle when we see someone nodding in front of the TV, at the movies, or during a political speech. Poor fella needs a vacation! we think, without much compassion. But sleep problems and sleep deprivation are no laughing matter. Sleep-challenged people are irritable, inattentive, and accident prone. They are more likely to suffer depression, heart disease, or stroke than their well-rested peers. A 1999 study reported in the journal *Sleep* notes that insomniacs suffer impaired concentration, impaired memory, a decreased ability to accomplish daily tasks, a decreased ability to enjoy interpersonal relationships, and an increased use of health care services. The *Archives of Internal Medicine* notes that insomnia sufferers are more likely to develop affective disorders, heart disease, and other adverse health outcomes. Another study puts it more bluntly: "Insomnia is predictive of cardiovascular and non-cardiovascular disease."

A study of the hormonal consequences of sleep deprivation was conducted by University of Chicago's Eve Van Cauter and associates at a Belgian university. They found that restricting sleep to four hours per night brings disturbance in the activity and timing of several important hormones including cortisol, melatonin, leptin, thyroid hormones, and prolactin. The study states, "Since these alterations are qualitatively and quantitatively similar to those observed during aging and sometimes during depression, a state of sleep debt, as is experienced by a substantial fragment of the population in modern societies, is likely to increase the severity of depression and widespread age-related chronic conditions such as obesity, diabetes, and hypertension."

Numerous studies associate insomnia with reduction in immune function. One, conducted at a German university, investigated measures of immune defense as well as subjective well-being and psychosocial performance in ten healthy males before and after sleep deprivation and again after recovery sleep. Sleep deprivation evoked not only decreased function of the immune system, most clearly visible on the morning following the sleepless night, but also deterioration of both mood and ability to work, which were most prominent the following evening.

The list of health consequences of insomnia goes on. It would take the rest of this book to detail all the negative health effects of sleep loss, though that is not our purpose here. Perhaps a monetary estimate will best suggest the full scope of the problem. According to one estimate, sleeplessness costs $15.9 billion a year in health care costs alone.

Accidents are another serious consequence of the insomnia epidemic. The National Highway Traffic Safety Administration (NHTSA) attributes over 100,000 automobile crashes per year to drowsy drivers, with 1,500 fatalities, 71,000 injuries, and a monetary cost of $12.5 billion. A British study revealed that drivers who report moderate to severe daytime sleepiness (about 20 percent of all drivers) are twice as likely to have been involved in a crash as other drivers. Yet 37 percent of respondents to an NHTSA poll said they have fallen asleep behind the wheel, 8 percent having done so in the last six months. But accidents don't occur only on the road. Do the names Bhopal, Chernobyl, and *Exxon Valdez* ring a bell? Sleep-deprived workers were implicated in each of these industrial disasters.

Insomnia plays no favorites either: our doctors, our police, our pilots, and our military personnel, all those charged with protecting our lives, are just as likely as the rest of us, perhaps more so, to suffer insomnia and sleep deprivation. Does it matter? Of course. Sleep deprivation wreaks havoc with our physical, cognitive, and intellectual abilities. One study of motor and sensory performance during and after experimentally induced sleep deprivation found a general reduction in overall response speed, a decrease in the speed of the fastest responses, and an increase in "lapsing"— delays in responding to stimuli—which in turn produced further decreases in response speed.

Mark Rosekind, a consultant for industrial sleep hygiene, says that many pilots, policemen, and doctors admit to making errors in sleep-deprived states of consciousness. According to his findings, cited in *Business Week,* 19 percent of health care workers report worsening a patient's condition because of fatigue; 44 percent of law enforcement officers report taking unnecessary risks while tired; and 80 percent of U.S. regional pilots say they've fallen asleep in the cockpit. William C. Dement, in his book *The Promise of Sleep,* describes tests Rosekind conducted on commercial pilots during long-haul flights between the West Coast and Japan. He found that pilots' reaction times during these prolonged flights often dropped 25 percent, and they frequently lapsed into "microsleeps" lasting five to ten seconds or more. These lapses of consciousness occurred not only in mid-flight but, even more alarmingly, during takeoffs and landings. A recent U.S. Army study suggests that combat stress and sleep deprivation may affect soldiers so badly that they perform as if they were drunk or sedated. Ill effects include slower reaction times, reduced vigilance, and problems remembering key details.

The bottom line? Estimates of the total monetary cost of insomnia and other sleep disorders, including medical, property damage, industrial accidents, employee absenteeism, and lost productivity, approach $45 billion per year. This is a huge cost for society to bear. But the human cost is far higher. Sleeplessness threatens our jobs, our relationships, and our health. It is a major public health issue that impacts the quality of life of millions of people.

On the Brighter Side

God bless the inventor of sleep, the cloak that covers all men's thoughts, the food that cures all hunger . . . the balancing weight that levels the shepherd with the king and the simple with the wise.

—MIGUEL DE CERVANTES,
Don Quixote

Now you know the dark side of sleep. Fortunately, there is a brighter side, too: Sleep, when we get the right quantity and quality of it, is nature's best medicine—a universal tonic that boosts our energy and vitality, elevates our mood, quells anxiety, and enhances our ability to learn and remember. When we are well rested, we're more at peace with the world around us and with our fellow human beings. We're more patient and compassionate. Recent research even indicates that sleep makes us smarter and more creative! But here no scientific data is really required, because anyone who has ever endured a string of sleepless nights and dragged through the days that follow them knows what a relief it is to awaken from that first, full night of blissful, restorative slumber. Suddenly the world seems to be a brighter, kinder, gentler place. We feel happier, stronger, and smarter. We feel more balanced and relaxed, more alert and alive.

Scientific research does confirm these subjective feelings about sleep. After centuries during which sleep was believed to be merely a quiescent state of brain and body, contemporary science is beginning to identify numerous, positive benefits conveyed by natural, restful sleep. In the brain, lower metabolic rates and brain temperatures during quiet sleep provide an opportunity for brain cells to recover from oxidative damage done by free radicals during waking hours. Most regions of the brain cannot regenerate cells as other organs do, so this sleep-dependent repair work is essential for keeping the brain in good working order. The active, or rapid eye movement (REM), phase of sleep, when we do most of our dreaming, brings a temporary cessation of release of the

essential neurotransmitters norepinephrine, serotonin, and hista-
mine. This brief respite, which comprises about 20 percent of
total sleep time, allows the receptors for these neurotransmitters
to rest, restoring them to their appropriate levels of sensitivity.
The restored sensitivity is thought to play an important role in
regulating mood during waking hours.

As we have seen, sleep deprivation depresses the functioning of
the immune system, but the converse is also true. A good night's
sleep has a wonderful restorative effect on our body's defense system. In one experiment, a group of nineteen healthy people were
given a hepatitis vaccination followed by either a full night of
sleep or a night of sleep deprivation. Four weeks later, the sleep
group exhibited nearly twofold higher hepatitis A virus (HAV)
antibody titer, indicating a considerably more robust immune
response.

Sleep is unquestionably the most effective stress-reduction
technique we will ever know. The demands of daily life can over-
charge the sympathetic branch of the autonomic nervous system,
triggering the so-called fight-or-flight mechanism that launches
mind and body into overdrive in response to stress and keeping it
there for prolonged periods. Sleep, particularly deep sleep, effectively rebalances the system, giving the parasympathetic branch,
which governs our ability to "rest and digest," a chance to assert
itself. In this way sleep moderates the effects of stress and switches
the body into self-healing mode.

Watching your weight? Deep, restful sleep is something you
can't do without, according to Van Cauter. Human growth hormone (HGH), which drives the growth of living tissue during
childhood, takes on the job of regulating weight, among other
functions, in adulthood. And HGH is secreted only during deep
sleep. Without sleep, even the most ardent weight watcher will
experience plenty of frustration but not much weight loss.

Can sleep really make you smarter or more skillful? It seems so. A large number of studies offer extensive evidence supporting this role of sleep in what is becoming known as sleep-dependent memory processing. These studies indicate that what we learn during waking hours requires distinct periods of consolidation before it is finally retained in our memories and reflected in our abilities. The simple passage of time does part of the job, but sleep has the unique capacity to enhance the process.

In one Harvard study, subjects trained in a finger-tapping task at either ten in the morning or ten in the evening were tested immediately following training and again twelve hours later without further training. The morning group, who had remained awake for the twelve hours following training, displayed modest gains in speed and accuracy of performance. But the evening group, who received a full night of sleep before the retest, scored startling performance gains averaging 20 percent for speed and 39 percent for accuracy as compared with the no-sleep group. Additional gains were seen over the following two nights. Similar results have been obtained in auditory and language learning tasks, visual texture discrimination tasks, and others.

Another study, conducted at the University of Lübeck in Germany and published in *Nature*, suggests that sleep brings insight, helping us to find creative solutions to difficult problems. In the study, 106 volunteers aged eighteen to thirty-two were asked to solve a "number reduction task" in which they could gradually improve their score by increasing their response speed with each round. However, they could also improve abruptly by gaining insight into a secret abstract rule underlying all the sequences. After initial exposure to the task, a third of the participants slept eight hours, another third were kept awake, while a third group was retested after eight hours of waking activities. Upon subsequent retesting, participants in the sleep group were twice as likely to discover the hidden rule as members of the other two groups. This research has great significance for both children's school performance as well as workplace productivity and creativity.

Want to excel in school or industry? Be sure to get plenty of sleep. Want a strong immune system? Sleep. Want vibrant good health, happiness, and a trim figure? Sleep, sleep, sleep.

Chronic insomnia and sleep disorders are medical problems, and therefore beyond the scope of this book. If you experience sleeplessness or other sleep-related symptoms for a week or more, ask your doctor or other medical provider to work with you to discover and alleviate the causes of your problem. Of course, once you've addressed all of the medical issues, you are welcome to return to these pages for help in restoring your natural, human ability to fall asleep and sleep through the night. What is presented here is applicable to anyone who wishes to learn how to encourage and amplify those natural, God-given processes that enable us to obtain the rest we need.

However, many people experience transitory insomnia with no apparent medical cause. They exhibit no diagnosable medical condition, other than an inability to sleep for one or several nights. The condition may come and go, it may disappear for a time, it may recur. That doesn't make it any less troubling! If that sort of transitory insomnia is what ails you, this book is for you! Dive right in, and you will learn what you need to know to fall asleep effortlessly at bedtime and to return to sleep quickly should you awaken during the night or early morning.

Stress: The Principal Cause of Insomnia

What causes the transitory insomnia that plagues so many millions of us? And more important, why is it happening to you? The short answer is, *stress*. Stress is the principal cause of insomnia. But what is stress? Everyone talks about stress, and everyone suffers from it at one time or another, but when we come right down to it, we're not really sure what stress is. So let's try to clarify it a bit.

Any healthy animal, whether it's a jellyfish, your family dog, or you, exists for most of its life in a state of homeostatic balance. That means that certain essential measures of vitality—fluid balance, caloric intake, temperature, and so on—are kept close to the ideal "set point." This allows the organism to function at its peak potential.

A *stressor* is anything that throws that fundamental balance out of whack, and *stress* is the variety of physical responses the organism uses in attempting to restore it. In human beings, the stress response begins with the release of two hormones from the adrenal glands: epinephrine and cortisol. These two hormones channel extra energy to the muscles and boost blood supply to allow quick action in response to the stressor. At the same time, they withdraw energy from processes that aren't needed for short-term survival, like growth and digestion.

The stress response is often triggered by an acute physical threat or demand—fleeing from a predator is the most often cited example—but it can also result from less dramatic factors such as heat or cold, scarcity of food or water, exposure to pollutants or toxins, immobilization, crowding, noise, darkness, and, yes, lack of sleep. Then there are such intangibles as fear, anger, grief, uncertainty, even extreme joy. All of these things are stressors; all of them are capable of provoking a stress response.

When the average animal encounters a stressor, its body produces a stress response for only as long as necessary and then returns quickly and efficiently to its previous homeostatic state. But humans and other primates are not your average animal. For them, the stress response can be triggered not only by real threats but also by the mere anticipation of one. Sometimes, if stressful events persist for a long time or recur with great frequency, or even if we just anticipate that they will, the stress response becomes a more or less permanent state of affairs.

When the stress response becomes the norm rather than a transitory state, then we are in for some real trouble. In the homeostatic state, our bodies conserve energy, using only what is necessary to maintain the balance of life. But with the stress response, there is a generalized increase in our metabolic rate: Our pulse quickens, our blood pressure and oxygen consumption soar, our muscles tense, and our body temperature runs hotter than normal, as if to prepare us for immediate action. But this is far more energy than we can afford to spend on a regular basis. Whereas the purpose of the stress response is to restore the body to balance, prolonged or unremitting stress creates serious imbalances of its own. Keeping all our bodily systems in a constant state of alarm eventually wears us out. It's no wonder that stress plays a role in the development of so many diseases, from heart attacks and stroke to anxiety and depression, diabetes, ulcers, colitis, and cancer.

So where does insomnia fit into this picture? How does stress cause insomnia? To understand that, we must first know a little bit about the physical processes that occur when we fall asleep. Falling asleep is a natural process that involves a distinct sequence of events in the body. As we approach sleep, there is a gradual lowering of metabolism. Our heart rate slows and our blood pressure declines. Our breathing becomes more regular, and we consume less oxygen. Our postural muscles, which have worked all day to keep us upright and moving about, now relax. At the same time, there are changes in the processing activity of the brain. The activity of neurons in the cerebral cortex becomes first slower, and then more synchronized, indicating a shift away from the complex, activated patterns of waking consciousness and toward a homogenous, deactivated state. As a result, we cease to process the sensory messages coming in from the outside world, and we slip into quiet sleep.

If we compare this description of the sleep-onset process to the description of the stress response in the preceding paragraph, it becomes very obvious that these are two antagonistic processes. Falling asleep involves a decrease in metabolism, and a gradual cessation of readiness for action, whereas the stress response involves a rapid increase in metabolism, sending the organism into a state of preparedness for action. The sleep process decreases arousal, making us less alert, while the stress response increases arousal, making us more so.

You'll remember we mentioned that the adrenal hormone cortisol was a trigger of the stress response. That's not cortisol's only job, however. In addition to the sharp transitory peaks of cortisol secretion that characterize the stress response, there is also a daily, cyclical rise and fall of cortisol levels that govern our level of wakefulness throughout the day and night. Cortisol is excitatory; it arouses us and wakes us up. Blood levels of cortisol have been shown to increase between 50 and 160 percent within thirty minutes of waking; that produces the powerful jolt of arousal needed to wake us up and get us moving in the morning. Then, cortisol levels decline as the day wears on and reach their lowest point in the evening, allowing us to rest, relax, and sleep.

But, as we know, cortisol levels can also be affected by the conditions of our daily existence. Dangerous, demanding, or threatening events—stressors—cause us to temporarily secrete higher levels of cortisol. That's a good thing, because we need to be aroused in order to answer the challenges that arise in the course of our lives. But when, as a result of prolonged or unremitting stress, whether real or perceived, our cortisol levels get stuck at a chronically higher level, that's bad news for our bodies and minds, and especially bad news for our ability to sleep and rest. Chronic over-secretion of cortisol leaves us chronically hyperaroused. Numerous studies indicate that insomnia is accompanied by excessive activation of the stress-response system not only during waking hours but during sleep as well. Furthermore, chronically elevated levels of cortisol and its precursor, adrenocorticotropic hormone (ACTH), can make sleep shallow, fragmented, and unrestful; delay the onset of sleep; and produce more frequent nocturnal awakenings.

To summarize: Stress is the principal cause of insomnia. Stress hormones are excitatory. When stress becomes chronic, we become chronically excited, or hyperaroused. When we're chronically hyper-aroused, we can't sleep, and the sleep we do get is not as restful.

The Big Question: How Much Sleep Do You Need?

This is the question I'm asked most frequently, and it's a tricky one. Each person's needs are different, not only for sleep but also for all aspects of life. Consequently, there are probably as many ways to answer the question as there are people! To approximate any kind of an answer I would need to know: What is your age? What is the state of your health? What are your personal sleep rhythms? What is your profession? What is your work schedule? What is most important to you in life? What are your dreams, your aspirations? What is your life's purpose? When we know all of that and more, we can see how sleep fits into the total picture, and we can start to come up with an individual answer. In my private practice, I often spend quite a bit of time helping my clients discover how to balance their needs for sleep, rest, and repose with all the other aspects of their lives.

Of course, I cannot give an individual answer for each reader. I have to say something general that will be helpful to each of you! So here goes.

Before Thomas Edison's invention of the lightbulb and the advent of artificial lighting, it is believed that Americans slept an *average* of 10 hours per night. Medical science currently recognizes *8.4 hours* of sleep per night as the average sleep requirement for general good health, though recognizing that some people can get along fine on an hour or two less whereas others need an hour or two more. I don't disagree with that general rule of thumb, but my perspective is a little different since I view sleep as not merely a medical matter but also a personal and spiritual one. My interest is not only in general health but in personal growth, pleasure, and self-healing as well.

It is my belief that we *need* something like eight hours of sleep per night, give or take an hour or two, *but we can use a whole lot more.* You see, I believe there are parts of each one of us in a state of profound un-rest, and these parts of ourselves require more than ordinary nightly sleep to be fully rested and fully healed.

To make an analogy with nutrition, we all know that there is a minimum daily requirement (MDR) set by the government for certain nutrients—vitamins A, C, and E, calcium, magnesium, and so forth. The MDR for a given nutrient is the amount you need to maintain general health. But, as you may be aware, these same nutrients can be taken in larger doses to enhance our overall vigor and vitality and, in the case of illness or injury, to support healing. The same goes for sleep.

That 8.4 hours, give or take two, is your MDR for "vitamin S," sleep. That's a medical necessity! Still, you can take higher doses of sleep to dig down into those deeper recesses of yourself that need resting, nurturing, and healing to help them to regain their full vitality, their full aliveness. These pleasurable, all-natural "sleep supplements" may include minutes or hours added to your usual bedtimes, as well as daytime naps, breaks, periods of deep relaxation, introspection, meditation, daydreaming, and anything else that helps you to maintain a more peaceful existence. All of the Mini-Moves™ presented in this book are designed to help you do just that.

The Other Big Question: How Many Hours Should You Spend in Bed?

People so often wonder how many hours of sleep they need, but they rarely think about how many hours it might take to get those hours. The question is one of efficiency: *How many hours does it take to get eight hours' sleep?* If you really think about it, you'll see that it takes considerably more than eight hours! Or, to put it another way, eight hours *in bed* is not the same thing as eight hours' *sleep.* Here's why: Let's say you go to bed at 11 p.m. and you plan to wake up at 7 a.m. In other words, you're planning to spend eight hours in bed. How much sleep will you get during those eight hours? Well, how long does it take you to fall asleep? Five minutes? Ten? Twenty? Or more? It is perfectly normal to experience some lag time between hitting the pillow and actually drifting off to sleep (scientists call this the *sleep latency period*). To be accurate, we really can't count that latency period as part of the sleep total. Subsequently, when you calculate how much sleep you've had, please do subtract that lag time from the eight hours you spend in bed.

Ask yourself whether you tend to have periods of wakefulness during the night. Do you observe a nightwatch, awakening to muse or meditate some time during the late night or early morning? That's normal, too, and it can be richly rewarding, but how much does it detract from your actual snooze time? Finally, what about the morning? Do you wake up ten, twenty, or thirty minutes before 7 a.m., just lying there, luxuriating in the waning moments of bedtime? That's an agreeable way to start the day!

When you calculate your sleep time, however, that gets subtracted from the total.

So let's say you spent twenty minutes drifting off, twenty for the nightwatch, and twenty minutes lying in the gold of dawn. There goes sixty minutes of sleep right there! You got into bed at 11 and you got out eight hours later, but you *slept* for only seven hours! The bottom line is, depending on your sleep style, it may take considerably longer than eight hours to get eight hours' sleep.

Of course, this is only an example, and your own sleep needs and your sleep schedule may vary considerably. For that reason, I strongly suggest that you perform a similar calculation for your own bedtime habits, and determine exactly how much sleep you actually get. You may be surprised! As a result, you may wish to adjust your sleep schedule, allowing more time in bed so you can get the rest you need. *Sleep on it!*

Sleep Medication: Cold Comfort

Sleeping pills are currently a $2 billion industry, and for the pharmaceutical industry that's just an appetizer. An article in *Business Week* cites industry estimates that the market will more than double, to $5 billion by 2010. "This is unquestionably one of the largest potential pharmaceutical markets in the world," opines pharmaceutical executive Gary A. Lyons, quoted in the *New York Times* (January 14, 2004). This rosy forecast is based on the finding that only 40 percent of insomnia sufferers have been diagnosed, and of those, only about half are receiving treatment; and fueled by the expectation that new drugs entering the market will work more reliably than existing preparations and find greater acceptance among consumers. Industry-sponsored public-opinion campaigns begun years ago engender the belief that drug treatment for insomnia is on the one hand medically necessary, and on

natural, safe, and unremarkable as taking an aspirin
.

... It's telling to note that a recent study conducted at the Harvard Medical School found that half a dozen sessions of cognitive-behavioral therapy (CBT) can do more to help a troubled sleeper than the top-selling sleeping pill. CBT is a form of talk therapy previously proven to be highly effective for depression. The therapy addresses the root causes of insomnia—stress, worry, fear, anxiety—and teaches the patient to handle them more effectively. To me, that seems a much safer and more appealing solution than drugs. And by the way, the deeply relaxing movement and breathing techniques presented in this book are completely compatible with all psychotherapeutic approaches. The therapy addresses the emotional and behavioral roots of your problem, whereas the movement techniques restore your inborn ability for natural, restful sleep. Of course, swallowing a single pill at bedtime would be quicker and require less attention on your part. But I think you're worth a little extra time and attention, especially when the end result is likely to be safer, better, and longer lasting.

I personally have no qualms about sleeping pills as a last resort. I'm glad they're available to folks who are enduring pain, illness, side effects of chemotherapy, or overwhelmingly stressful life events, and who would otherwise go sleepless for long periods. In those cases I consider sleep medication to be a blessing. Why should people suffer when medications can help? However, sleep medication has become the first, rather than the last, resort even for short-term, transitory insomnia. "Missed a couple nights' sleep?" say our doctors with increasing frequency, "here's a sample. Take as needed."

It's easy to start on sleeping pills, but it's not always easy to stop. Much of my private practice consists of people who are terribly eager to wean themselves off sleeping pills, most of them in the grip of a single best-selling brand. They welcomed sleeping pills as an easy ride to sounder sleep, and now they find they can't get off the merry-go-round. Although they may not be technically "habituated," they may struggle with "rebound insomnia," sleeplessness that results when sleep drugs are withdrawn. After a period in which the sleep-wake rhythm was controlled by a drug rather than the body's natural timekeeping mechanisms, it can be hard for mind and body to resume their former duties. Even if you're suffering rebound insomnia, don't despair! If you're truly committed to your own self-healing, the insomnia solution presented in this book can help you.

If you're considering trying sleeping pills, here are four questions I suggest you ask your doctor—and yourself. First, how will sleeping pills affect sleep quality? Is the sleep you get with a pill equivalent to the natural, restful sleep we were born to enjoy? Or is it just an imitation of the real thing, like coffee creamer or a Dynel hairpiece? Bear in mind, sleep is more than just becoming unconscious for eight hours. Just as a balanced meal contains all the essential nutrients in precise proportion, natural sleep contains all the essential stages of sleep in precise proportion, too. Disturb that essential balance of sleep, as many medications are known to do, and you may get something quite different. What does modern science say on the subject? Is there any research to guide you? Sadly, not much. Research takes lots of money, and most studies on sleeping drugs are funded by the manufacturers themselves. They are interested in how long a drug takes to act, how long its effects last, and what the side effects are. That's about as far as it goes.

Second, what are the long-term effects of sleeping pill use? Sleeping pills can't actually cure insomnia. They are at best a stopgap solution designed to tide you over until the causes of the problem abate. Note that no sleeping pill has ever been tested or approved for more than short-term use—a month at best. Yet many troubled sleepers take them for months or even years. What are the health effects? What are the consequences? We can't be certain.

Third, how long will the drug retain its effectiveness? Many sleeping pills work one way when you start, and quite differently a month or two later. Your body and mind may become desensitized to the drug's effect. You might need to add another drug, and then another, just to get the same effect you began with. Not a few people end up taking several drugs, every night at bedtime, without a cure in sight. I have clients who take three different sleep medications every night; in *The Promise of Sleep,* Dement reports patients who take as many as *eight.*

Fourth, what's the exit strategy? How long should you plan to use this drug, and what will it take for you to stop? Will you experience rebound insomnia? Please discuss these and any other questions you may have with your doctor or other health care provider before embarking on a course of sleep medication. With your doctor's consultation, and a bit of your own research, you can make the decision that's right for you.

Even if you do decide to go the medication route, I hope you will choose to learn the gentle sleep-inducing exercises in this book as well. They will make your daily life more peaceful, thereby hastening the day when you won't need sleeping pills anymore. And when that day comes, the gentle, synchronized movements and breathing will put the healing power of natural, restful sleep quite literally at your fingertips.

The "Sleep Switch" and How to Flip It

More than seventy years ago, a gifted neurologist named Constantin van Economo speculated that there were physical structures in the brain that were responsible for sleep and waking. He postulated a wakefulness center in the posterior hypothalamus and a sleep-promoting center in the preoptic area. Twenty years later, a Dutch neurologist, Nauta, discovered that an incision in the front of a rat's hypothalamus interfered with its ability to sleep and one in the back of the hypothalamus sent it into a coma. But the exact location and character of the neurons responsible were unknown.

Recently, building on these earlier discoveries, a team at Harvard Medical School has located two centers in the rat brain, which they believe constitute the "sleep switch" in the human brain. As predicted, the ventrolateral preoptic nucleus (VLPO) in the front of the hypothalamus contains neurons that are active during sleep, while the posterior lateral hypothalamus contains neurons that are crucial for maintaining normal wakefulness. It seems that these two centers carry on an ongoing neurological tug-of-war in which each center attempts to inhibit, or suppress, the other's activity. Whether we're awake or asleep at any given moment depends on which of these centers is dominant at the time. Taken together, these interdependent structures are said to constitute a sleep switch that, when functioning properly, keeps us awake during the day and asleep through the night. By the same token, disruption of the communicating pathway between the two structures may be a cause of insomnia and other sleep disorders. Reports of these discoveries have caused a stir in the media, even making it to the cover of *Newsweek*. Much of the excitement centers on the search for new sleep drugs. Now that they think they know where the sleep switch is located, scientists plan to invent new drugs that will allow us to flip it "on" whenever we like. The hope is that the new drugs, rather than sedating the entire central nervous system, might act more specifically on the centers that actually control sleep, providing something closer to natural, restful slumber than existing sleep preparations, without the side effects, potential drug dependency, and unpredictable results.

My response to the discovery of the alleged sleep switch is a bit different. I welcome the discovery as a scientific elucidation of something I already know in my own experience. For I have known for some time how to flip the sleep switch without drugs, without any artificial aids whatsoever. And I can teach it to you, too. Using the simple, immediately available tools of physical movement and breathing, you can learn to throw the sleep switch whenever you need to. In doing so, you needn't introduce any foreign substances into your body. Rather, you can switch on your body's innate faculty for healthy, restful sleep simply by acting in perfect accord with nature's laws and your own deepest needs. And it won't cost a penny. That's what we're going to talk about in the next chapters.

Chapter 1

Profiles in Sounder Sleep

> "Good-bye sleep lab, hello Sounder Sleep System! After working the night shift for twenty years my brain couldn't tell night from day. Now I sleep like a baby lamb."
> —J.P., *IT officer*

Janet is an editor for a local news organization. It's late morning, about time for a coffee break. After a morning of fast-paced newsroom action, Janet's body feels tense, her skull seems to be pulsating, and her mind is racing. Instead of heading for the coffee cart, Janet puts her three computers to sleep, activates her voice mail, and lowers her hands to her lap. Joining her hands, she closes her eyes and rests quietly. Her breathing becomes slower and softer. Each time she inhales, Janet gradually twists and bends her wrists slightly so that the knuckles of both hands rise gently toward the ceiling. Each time she exhales, her wrists relax and the hands come to rest in her lap. Often she pauses for a few breaths, then continues. After five minutes Janet slowly opens her eyes, breathes what appears to be a deep sigh of relief, and heads down the hall for a cup of herbal tea. Her eyes are twinkling, her mind is calm and clear, her energy is renewed.

Tim is a recently retired executive in good health, enjoying newfound freedom from the corporate grind. It's 3 a.m., and he has slept soundly since he and his wife, Maggie, turned in at

> "I'm just amazed. Sleep is no longer a problem for me!"
> —BILL H., *fibromyalgia sufferer*

11:30. He's just made a quick trip to the bathroom and returned to bed. But now he's awake. Eager to return to sleep quickly and efficiently, Tim takes action. He lightly touches the tip of his tongue to a spot on the inside of his cheek. With each inhalation he pushes gently outward against the elastic tissues of his cheek. With each exhalation he allows his tongue to relax. After six or seven repetitions of that modest movement, he stops to rest. After a few minutes, his jaw becomes slack, his breathing gets a little fuller, and his mind is occupied with dreamlike thoughts. Soon he and Maggie are sleeping peacefully again, side by side.

Abby suffers from fibromyalgia, a chronic pain syndrome of unknown cause. Sufferers feel pain at certain "tender points" on the neck, shoulders, back, and hips. Insomnia and un-restful sleep are among the symptoms associated with the syndrome. At bedtime, Abby lies on her right side, slowly moving her left hip downward in a series of steplike movements. The movements are light, easy, and soothing. After a few minutes of that Abby rests quietly, tuning in to the calming effect of the movement. Another round of movements, another pause, and Abby drifts off to sleep.

Later that night, around 2 a.m., Abby wakes up again for no apparent reason. She's feeling vaguely anxious and her body is sore, as is typical of fibromyalgia sufferers. Rolling to her side, she repeats the same sequence of gentle movements she did at bedtime, pausing frequently to rest and feel the effects. Within minutes, Abby's anxiety has lost its edge and the soreness has abated. Abby drifts back to sleep.

What are Janet, Tim, and Abby doing? Is it some sort of meditation? Yes and no. Exercises? Well, not exactly. In fact they are practicing Mini-Moves, gentle, synchronized movements and breathing, alternating with periods of quiet rest. Mini-Moves are the basic building blocks of the Sounder Sleep System™, a practical, innovative system of self-healing for insomnia and the stress of life.

During waking hours these gentle, natural Mini-Moves relieve physical tension and help you stay calm, even under stress. At bedtime, they help you relax your body, calm your mind, and lull yourself into a blissful, restorative slumber. If you wake during the night, these same Mini-Moves help you get back to sleep fast.

Just like Janet or Tim or Abby, you, too, can benefit from these unique techniques. Thousands of people in North America and Europe have already learned the Mini-Moves from a nurse, physical therapist, counselor, or other healing-arts practitioner and experienced the benefits. In the pages that follow, you will learn how to do the Mini-Moves yourself, and how to make them a part of your life. Once you've learned the basics, you can do them anytime, anywhere to rest and recover from the stress of life and to achieve more restful sleep.

Used regularly and conscientiously in conjunction with some commonsense lifestyle guidelines, these gentle, pleasurable techniques can be your surest ally in your struggle against insomnia and the stress of life. As a result, your life will get sweeter and more peaceful. Your thoughts will become more positive, your creativity will flourish, and you'll see a happier, healthier, and more energetic person in the mirror.

Does that sound good to you? Great! Everything you need to know is right in this book. Read on!

The Eternal Quest: Self-Healing Then and Now

From our very beginnings, we humans have been engaged in a quest for self-healing. Whenever we were ill, injured, sleepless, or afraid, we looked for resources in our own environment that we could use to recover our full health and vitality. These resources included healing foods and medicines derived from plants, animals, and the earth; healing prayer, meditation, ritual, singing, and chanting; rest cures and pilgrimages to sacred sites; and an endless variety of human-centered means of healing, employing touch, mindful movement, and breath. This self-healing tradition goes back as far as we care to look.

The common herb yarrow, known to modern botanists as *Achillea millefolium,* gives us clear proof of the historical continuity of the self-healing quest. Fossilized yarrow pollen has been discovered in caves occupied by the Neanderthal people over sixty thousand years ago. This same herb appears in ancient Greek mythology; it is said that Achilles (for whom the herb appears to be named) gave it to his soldiers during the battle of Troy to stop the bleeding of their wounds. The Navajos considered yarrow a panacea, a cure for all ills, and this was echoed by English traditional herbalists, who called it an "allheal" herb. Early American settlers used it for urinary problems, head colds, and more.

Consider another timeless self-healing practice—chanting. It has existed in one form or another in virtually every human culture. The Vedic sages of India employed chanting to purify the mind and body over five thousand years ago, and their methods are still used today. Sufis, the Middle Eastern mystical sect best known for the "whirling dervishes," trace their healing chants back "to the time of Adam." And Alfred A. Tomatis, a medical doctor who has made pioneering studies of the neurophysiology of sound, extols the virtues of the millennium-old Gregorian chant for promoting and restoring health, energy, and vitality. He believes that the high frequencies of the tenor voices "charge" the nervous system while the slow, breath-paced rhythms lead to a relaxed heart rate. The result is a state Tomatis calls "body relaxed/mind alert," which he deems ideal for learning and healing.

These few examples of healing chants are by no means all-inclusive. The Africans, Greeks, Romans, Native Americans, Mayans, Jews, and many other peoples have employed chants in combined spiritual-religious and healing practices. Chanting, the prolonged, repetitive singing of sacred words or syllables, uses the most elemental means available for healing—the human body itself. Chanting is a powerful healing practice that engages voice, breath, physical movement, and mind in a vigorous, well-coordinated, rhythmic action. In addition to its spiritual functions, chanting has the potential to induce rapid, positive change at many levels of being, including blood pressure, immune function, posture, mood, and more. Chanting can even be used to induce sleep!

And consider yoga, the ancient Indian system of exercises for health and well-being that has taken the country by storm, breaking out of its niche as an esoteric spiritual practice to feature prominently on the covers of national magazines like *Vogue* and *Time,* the latter declaring it to be a "75 million dollar a year industry." But yoga is far more than just the physical-fitness flavor of the month. In the nearly two-thousand-year-old *Yoga-Sûtra,* attributed to Patanjali, the physical postures of yoga are considered not as an end in themselves, but as a means for balancing, healing, and strengthening the human body in preparation for a comprehensive program for the liberation of the spirit. "Yoga," declares Patanjali, "is the cessation of the fluctuation of the mind." But the yogic system predates Patanjali, probably by eons. Its origins lie in the native self-healing culture of the Indian subcontinent, in which the ever-available medium of movement and breath, along with medicinal herbs, massage, diet, and natural hygiene practices, constituted a cutting-edge self- and community-care technology. Analogous healing systems appear in China, Tibet, Korea, Southeast Asia, Polynesia, and the Middle East, invariably intermixed with the indigenous philosophy and religion: Hinduism, Buddhism, Sufism, Taoism, Bön, and so forth. In those philosophies, God, Heaven, Nature, Man, Body, and Breath were not piecemeal entities such as we conceive them, but were understood to be multiple expressions of a single, supreme unifying principle. Healing the ills of the body was seen as a process of alignment or harmonization with this primal force in all of its manifestations.

The martial arts of China, India, and Japan reveal another historical root of the self-healing project. The arts we know today as karate, jiujitsu, kung fu, and many others were founded by warriors who, ever at risk for bodily hurt and harm, had to be masters of the simplest, most effective, ready-to-hand means of healing wounds, sprains, fractures, hemorrhage, poisoning, and the like. This was a matter of sheer survival. To that end, manual manipulation, movement, and breath techniques were key components of the martial artist's *materia medica*. Vestiges of those healing practices persist, often unrecognized or only vaguely acknowledged, in the practice of modern martial arts, and they remain explicit in the "soft" martial art taiji, in qigong, and related Taoist practices. Recently we have seen a resurgence of so-called medical qigong used, often with doctors' consent and encouragement, as an adjunct to Western medical treatment.

Clearly, self-healing occupies an important place in human history. It reflects the ageless need of human beings to care for ourselves *with whatever means are at our disposal,* whether it is the clay under our feet, the plants in the forests, or the very air that we breathe. And this self-healing tradition is still alive and well, though perhaps no longer considered the mainstream of medical care. Even so, we tend to forget it, or minimize its importance. We forget that there was a time when for most people the nearest doctor or clinic might have been hundreds of miles away, and people had to know how to heal themselves. We forget that there was an even earlier time when there were no doctors or clinics at all, and then people *really* had to know how to heal themselves. And we forget, or fail to notice, that, as we shall see, self-healing is going on all the time, right under our noses.

So, how do we approach self-healing for insomnia and the stress of life? What are the basic components of this self-healing system? That will be revealed as this chapter unfolds.

The Spirit of Self–Healing

These ancient philosophies and practices of self-healing have always held great appeal for me. At an early age I studied martial arts, then meditation, then massage, healing foods, taiji, and qigong, and I continue to pursue these studies to this day. I have known many fine teachers who strongly influenced my thinking, several of whom will be acknowledged as we proceed. For now, there is one in particular I'd like to mention because his message relates to the core philosophy, to the spirit, of the insomnia solution presented in this book.

About ten years ago I had the good fortune to attend a series of lectures given by Michel Abehsera, a longtime teacher of natural healing. At the time, Abehsera used to bill himself as a "savant, raconteur, and bon vivant," and he was all of that, and more. Despite their serious themes, his lectures had the form and feel of rambling folktales, with an engaging, humorous quality that made it easy to take in his message. These made a profound impression on me and contributed greatly to my understanding of the self-healing process.

By heritage a Moroccan Jew, Abehsera was one of the first American students of Japanese health guru George Ohsawa, who in the early 1960s introduced America to such esoteric food items as brown rice and pesticide-free, organically grown vegetables, as well as shiatsu massage and acupuncture. At the time, these seemed rather cultish, even freaky. Today, of course, many of these innovations are widely known and accepted. In this period Abehsera wrote several best-selling books of natural recipes, each one infused with a healthy measure of Eastern philosophy. But somewhere along the way he chucked the Eastern bit altogether and went back to his roots in Judaism. There he found the writings of Maimonides, the twelfth-century Hebrew physician and sage, on which he based his own distinctive approach to natural health and healing. Good-bye brown rice and seaweed, hello bread and olives!

Two of Abehsera's teaching tales bear repeating here, because they were my introduction to certain principles that are fundamental to the insomnia solution that you are about to learn. In one, he recalled how one of his cooking students had proudly presented him with an extracurricular "vegetarian pot pie" made of grains, vegetables, beans, nuts, seaweed, and seeds baked in a whole wheat crust. Despite its abundance of "healthy" ingredients, Abehsera explained, this turgid concoction was arguably inedible and definitely indigestible. Recalling how he had gently refused the proffered pie, Abehsera offered this as an illustration of the self-healing principle, "Don't punish yourself." By that he meant that whatever you do to nurture your own well-being, to heal yourself, must be light, easy, sweet, and pleasurable. Otherwise, you are just punishing yourself. And punishing yourself won't help. It only causes more suffering.

Another of Abehsera's stories harkened back to a time in the early 1960s when he was building the Paradox, probably the first natural-food restaurant in New York City. (Nowadays there are dozens of them, in some cases two or three on the same block!) He was so immersed in the design and construction of his new restaurant that he didn't have time to meet with all the people who were calling him for health consultations. Eventually, Abehsera recalled, "whatever complaint people had, I told them, 'Take barley soup!' And you know," he said with an impish twinkle in his eye, "it worked!" The idea here was that self-healing needn't involve elaborate means or exotic substances, and needn't rely on the powerful effects (and the attendant side effects!) that we have come to expect from pharmaceuticals. Oftentimes something as simple, earthy, and readily available as barley soup can be enough to jump-start our innate faculty for self-healing. That means that wherever we are, whether it's a high-rise building in a big city, a shack in the middle of the desert, or a boat on the ocean, there is bound to be *something* at hand that we can use to heal ourselves.

Years went by, and I hardly gave a thought to Abehsera and his oddly entrancing tales. But those two principles of his had somehow wormed their way into the depths of my consciousness: first, that pleasure—not punishment—is our first, best ally in self-healing; and second, that often the safest, most effective medicine is something to be found right at our fingertips. These principles were to serve me well when I found myself in dire need of self-healing.

My Quest for Sounder Sleep

Several years ago I had a major bout of insomnia. I was going through a difficult time in my life, with several big upheavals happening all at once: one of those midlife crises you hear people talk about. You hear about it and perhaps you think, It won't happen to me. Well, it did.

It was like this: After a busy day of juggling the mountain of seemingly insurmountable personal problems that was then my life, I'd get myself in bed by 10:30 or 11, and I'd fall asleep within fifteen minutes or so. So far, so good. But just a few hours later, around 2 or 3 a.m., *zing!*, my eyes would pop open like a couple of automotive airbags. This sudden awakening was accompanied by a rush of sensation in the pit of my stomach, a potent mix of anxiety, dread, and fear. The effect was like suddenly gulping down several cups of strong coffee (black, three sugars!). I was *wide* awake. And I felt completely helpless to do anything about it.

Once awake, I'd stay that way for two or three hours. Sometimes I'd lie in the dark, brooding about my personal problems (including, of course, my inability to sleep). Sometimes I'd read novels, magazines, or professional journals. Occasionally I'd pace the floor. On a good night, I'd meditate or do qigong, the Taoist self-healing exercises I'd studied on and off for the preceding fifteen years. Meditation and qigong calmed me considerably, but not enough to let me sleep. Only toward morning, as rosy-fingered dawn touched the rooftops of New York's upper west side, would I drift into a fitful sleep.

A scant hour or so later, with the sun in all its glory and the trucks on Columbus Avenue beginning their relentless daily rumble, the night was palpably over. I would tally up the anxious hours. "Let's see," I'd silently calculate, "to bed at 11, asleep by 11:15, woke up at 3. That's three hours and forty-five minutes of shut-eye. Then three hours of wakefulness. Back to sleep at six for an hour, maybe an hour and a quarter." I'd add the two blocks of sleep together to figure my total elapsed sleep time: five hours by the most liberal reckoning. Not nearly enough. I knew that I needed at least seven and a half hours just to feel alert and alive, and an hour more than that for full vitality and peak performance at my work. That's the way I'm made.

This went on for a week and more. Some nights were a little better, some were worse, but the cumulative effect was undeniable. My vital energy was being gradually depleted; I was beginning to drag through my days. And while I lived on the seventh floor, high enough above street level to enjoy an expansive view of city and sky, my mood dwelt somewhere below the sub-basement. Sound familiar?

Finally, I saw a doctor—because one *should* in such a case. He examined me, reviewed my history, and didn't seem overly concerned. In response to my request for a sleep aid, something "not too heavy," he wrote a prescription for a pill with a name that sounded like a recreational drug from the '60s. Recreational it was not—aside from keeping me awake all night, it caused my eyes to cross, replaced my stride with a stagger, and generally scared the daylights out of me. Later, I discovered that this was no mere sleeping pill, but an antidepressant that is often prescribed in cases of depression accompanied by insomnia. "Not too heavy," indeed! Anyway, that was the end of sleeping pills for me. I was determined to find the natural way.

Questioning

Some nights later, lying in bed, staring at the ceiling, I began to form a question in my mind. I was into clean living—pure foods, regular exercise, organically grown foods, vitamins and minerals—anything I could do to take good care of my body. Not only that, but I also had been a student of modern and traditional self-healing methods since high school. What's more, I was by profession a teacher of the *Feldenkrais Method*®, the world-renowned system of "movement education" that employs gentle, guided body movements to encourage greater ease and spontaneity of thought, action, and expression. My mission was teaching people to use mindful, physical movement as the key to an easier, more pleasurable, and productive life. Even so, in spite of all my personal study, professional training, and long experience with self-healing, I could not summon a single technique that would help me sleep. Nowhere in my studies of taiji, qigong, yoga, or meditation had anyone said to me, "This is what you do to help yourself sleep when you can't."

Of course, there was no shortage of techniques to relax the body and calm the mind during waking hours, thereby making sleep more likely at bedtime. I had long been diligent in my daily practice of the Feldenkrais self-help method called Awareness Through Movement® (dubbed ATM for short—long before the advent of today's ever-present automated teller machines). Among the many benefits of ATM is its power to relieve physical stress and promote a state of profound mental and physical ease that is undoubtedly a valuable aid to sleep. You will find several Feldenkrais-flavored movement experiments in chapter 3 of this book. If excess physical tension is a strong component of your sleepless nights, that's a great place to start.

A good friend and long-experienced yoga teacher recommended as an adjunct to my personal ATM practice a sequence of yoga poses for me to practice during the day. They were wonderfully relaxing and helped me to center and stabilize my mind. In addition, one of my qigong teachers taught me some special exercises said to encourage deeper sleep. They were helpful, too. The more I did, the better I felt.

At this time, my apartment was half a block from Central Park, and like thousands of other New Yorkers, I put the park's well-paved drives to good use for vigorous physical exercise, particularly during the glorious weekend hours when they were closed to traffic. My favorite athletic pursuit was in-line skating, and I loved to do a vigorous lap around the long, looping drive that circles the park. I'd enter at Mariner's Gate on West 85th Street, zoom down the hill with the American Museum of Natural History to my right, under the perpetually stern gaze of Daniel Webster, immortalized in bronze at the 72nd Street crossover (LIBERTY AND UNION, NOW AND FOREVER, ONE AND INSEPARABLE.). From there I'd zip downtown, parallel to Central Park West.

So far, it had been mostly high-speed, downhill. But at the southeastern corner of the park the terrain begins to tilt the other way, and I would have to claw my way back up the east side, past the closely ranked mansions on Fifth Avenue and the giant, concrete corkscrew that is the Guggenheim Museum. By the time I reached 103rd Street, I'd be breathing pretty hard, so I'd most often take advantage of the convenient crossover there, thus avoiding the long hill leading into the upper reaches of the park. Even so, it was a great workout, and I believe that at age forty-eight I was in the best physical condition I'd ever known.

Why am I telling you this? Because, if you suffer from insomnia, you should know that physical fitness is one absolutely essential component of your personal insomnia solution. If you have even occasional insomnia, please do exercise wherever, whenever you can, whether that means walking a couple of miles to work, climbing stairs instead of riding the elevator, swimming laps at your local pool, or pumping iron at your local gym. Vigorous exercise lifts your spirits, puts a spring in your step, and makes your eyes sparkle in a way that makes you look younger than your years. And numerous studies show that vigorous exercise at any time of day—except in the evening, when exercise-induced stress hormone production can delay the onset of sleep—is one of the most effective lifestyle modifications you can make to promote natural restful sleep.

So there it is. I was doing all the right things to help myself sleep. Even so, in spite of my commitment to healthy food, supplements, Feldenkrais, yoga, qigong, and in-line skating, when that uninvited 3 a.m. wake-up call sounded, I was stumped. "Oh, shoot! What do I do now?" Sure, I could get out of bed and do some more Feldenkrais, yoga, or qigong, but in the process I would have to open my eyes and move my body, and that would likely wake me up even more. Besides, I didn't want to get out of bed. I needed rest, not more exercise! I needed something I could do right there in my bed to lull myself back to sleep.

There must be something I can do for myself, I thought. And there was. I remembered certain movements that I had learned fifteen years earlier during the period of my professional training, movements that had almost instantly overcome my resolve to play the alert, attentive student, sending me into a deep sleep right there on the floor of the training hall. I remembered only the first few movements in the sequence, and then waking up at the end of the class feeling wonderfully refreshed, if a little sheepish at having slept through class. (Later, I copied someone's notes so I would know what happened while I dozed!)

In a recently released transcript of that lesson as it was taught by Feldenkrais himself, entitled "Work with the Active [dominant] Hand," the Israeli movement master elaborates a sequence of exquisitely slow, gradual movements of the wrist, then the fingers, then the arm and shoulder. From the beginning of the lesson, he repeatedly exhorts his listeners to bend and straighten their wrists "slowly, slowly, with the greatest 'slowness' possible." By doing the movement "truly slowly, slowly," he insists, in his usual enigmatic way, "you will notice many things that you do not know." He was right about that. I did not know it at the time, but those "truly slow" movements and others like them would indeed bring me unexpected, and very welcome, insight.

At the time, I had considered those soporific Feldenkrais movements little more than a curiosity, but now, in my desperate search for a natural, drug-free insomnia solution, I wondered: Maybe those "truly slow" movements, or others like them, could be used to overcome insomnia. I began to recall other sleep-inducing ATM lessons as well, including an extended series taught over the course of several days in Dr. Feldenkrais's professional training program at Amherst in the summer of 1981 that are known simply as "the Bell Hand." Those had produced a profound tranquilizing effect whenever I'd done them. And it wasn't just me. Dozens of Feldenkrais's Amherst trainees had nodded off during those lessons.

An idea that now seems completely self-evident to me was just beginning to form in my mind, and it was this: Just as certain fast, vigorous movements—jumping jacks, for example—are known to be stimulating and invigorating, certain slow, gentle movements could be profoundly tranquilizing to the mind and to the body. And maybe, just maybe, I speculated, such profoundly tranquilizing movements could help you get to sleep and stay that way, even when your mind and body were crying, "Wake up!" I began to explore this idea in earnest.

The Breath Connection

I'm not going to tell you that my experiments were an instant success. Insomnia held me in its grip. But with a few weeks of persistent experimentation, and several seemingly fortuitous flashes of insight, I started to see the darkness at the end of the tunnel. (Yes, there was light there, too, but for now it was darkness and the bliss of natural sleep that I craved.) I continued to experiment with slow, gentle movements of the hand, wrist, and fingers alternating with periods of quiet rest.

At first I practiced more or less as Dr. Feldenkrais had taught, but I soon began to vary the movements, and the manner in which they were performed, to suit my own very specific purposes. You see, the Feldenkrais Method offers a very broad, practical program of self-discovery and personal growth. There is a lifetime of learning, and more, in those lessons of Moshe's. But right now I only wanted to learn one thing: to sleep through the night. So, instead of sticking to the strict Feldenkrais lessons, I started to tinker around with the movements in hopes of making them more specifically sleep inducing.

I experimented with other kinds of movements, too, some that were derived from my studies of taiji and qigong, and others that just seemed to come to me of their own accord, seemingly out of thin air. Whatever I did, I did "truly slowly" and with minimal, minimal force, often so slow and soft that the movements would have been undetectable to any casual observer. These exquisitely slow, gentle movements had a deeply calming effect on me, although in my sleep-disturbed state they alone were not yet enough to get me back on the sleep track. There were two additional pieces that had to fall into place before I would experience the full power of these techniques to relax my body, calm my mind, and lull me to sleep.

The first was to *synchronize my physical movements with the inflow and outflow of my breath*. The second was to punctuate those periods of synchronized movement and breathing with *extended periods of quiet rest*. For me, these two principles were the bridge between the canonical Feldenkrais movements, which were inherently relaxing but not necessarily sleep inducing, and a new and different quality of movement that would reliably deliver me to the shores of sleep, allowing me to get the rest I so needed. These gentle sleep-inducing techniques, wh come to call Mini-Moves, all employ the same basic components: *slow, gentle, physical movements synchronized with easy, natural breathing, alternating with extended periods of quiet rest.* These are the raw materials of which our insomnia solution is made.

First Results

The first sleep-inducing Mini-Move to really take shape for me was something I was to call "Breath Surfing" (presented in full detail in chapter 5). I used to practice it every night at bedtime, and then again if and when I awakened during the night. To begin, I'd place my hands on my upper chest and follow the rising and falling movements of the breath with my fingertips. Simply monitoring the movements of my own breath in that way seemed to have a distinctly calming effect. Later, I'd add very gentle, voluntary movements of my thumbs, synchronizing the movements with the rising and falling of my chest. Unaccountably, those gentle, synchronized movements seemed to cause my breath to become even slower and softer. I could feel how my pulse, which tends to be on the high side after an active day, would slow down as well. My whole body, legs, arms, lips, forehead, would become very still and quiet. As my body began to slow down, so did my mind. Little by little, my thoughts would relinquish their usual jackrabbit pace, becoming synchronized with the slow, steady rhythm of my breath. Occasionally, I'd stop and rest, just lying still and thinking of nothing in particular.

After several minutes of this, I'd find myself lapsing into a sleepy, dreamy, drowsy state that was neither deep sleep nor full waking, but rather a happy amalgam of the two. The movements of my thumbs would come to a halt; whether it was the result of my own drowsiness, or theirs, I knew not. There, behind my closed lids, against a velvety black curtain of darkness, I'd see brightly colored particles flowing in an endless stream, like luminous confetti. Later, these would give way to veils of pure, liquid color and dreamlike thoughts—images, associations, fragments of sentences that had neither the narrative coherence nor the emotional power of deep, sleeping dreams, but were nonetheless quite unlike rational, waking thought. At times, I would lapse back into something more like wakefulness, and I'd find myself thinking, Now I am awake! But this did not concern me, because I had come to understand that such brief moments of increased arousal were not the final, irrevocable waking of insomnia. They were only temporary switchbacks on the long and winding path that meanders from waking to sleep. Awakening like that, I'd resume the gentle movements of my thumbs, and in a few moments, I'd feel myself drifting once again in the direction of deep repose, relaxation, and sleep. Soon enough, that gentle drifting awareness would give way to the blissful unknowingness of natural, restful sleep.

Incidentally, the name Breath Surfing stems from my own lifetime passion for the sport of surfing. What's the connection? Most nonsurfers see a wave as a mass of water rolling in toward the shore. But surfers know that waves, even very large ones, move very little water toward the beach. What we call an "ocean wave" isn't so much moving water as it is an invisible, oscillating wave of kinetic energy moving through a water medium. Most of that energy is whipped up by gale-force winds near the Arctic Circle in winter and Antarctica in the summer. Those nascent waves then travel thousands of miles in deep, open water, are shaped and funneled by the islands, bays, channels, trenches, and banks they pass along the way, and finally break on the shallow reefs, rocks, and sandbars where surfers eagerly await their arrival. Thus the surfer who snakes his way across the face of a wave enters into an ecstatic pas de deux with the pure, elemental energies of air, water, and earth. This watery dance evokes a profound communion between his or her body and Mother Nature. Surfing may look extreme, but it is a very spiritual pursuit! And I believe that the continuous, rhythmic ebb and flow of the breath, and the invisible life-energy that drives it, have much that same quality, and a common origin. Hence the name. In surfing, we ride a wave of energy to the beach. In Breath Surfing, we ride a wave of energy to the shores of sleep.

As a result of these early experiments in Breath Surfing and related techniques, sleep and I were beginning to enjoy a far more cordial relationship than we had in a long time. True, most nights I was still waking up at 3 a.m., but my awakenings had a completely different quality. No longer did my eyes suddenly pop open; it was a much more gentle and gradual process. And instead of hours of unbidden wakefulness, it would now be just minutes—thirty, then fifteen, then five and less. As a result, my feelings of anxiety, fear, and dread gave way first to mild annoyance, then to indifference, and finally to delight. *So what* if I awakened at 3 a.m.? I had discovered that I could reliably get myself back to sleep in a relatively short time. This gave me tremendous confidence and hope. The feelings of helplessness were gone, too. That made sense, since I no longer *was* helpless. Instead of lying in bed waiting for sleep to come, I now had something I could *do*. With gentle, soothing, synchronized movements and breath I could invite sleep to come, and then welcome it with open arms.

A Second Stream

Around this time, something else happened that gave my investigation into the psychophysical mechanisms of sleep a welcome push in the right direction. I am a fairly solitary person, happiest working alone, or one-on-one with individual clients. I've been this way all my life. (Believe it or not, I dropped out of kindergarten after two weeks because I found it just too noisy, crowded, and stressful!) But I had a big promotional project on my hands just then, and I needed help, so I recruited a team of friends as assistants and set them to work. I was very grateful for their help and support, but was clear from the first that this solitary-leaning fellow was not cut out to be a team manager! The hubbub of several other souls occupying my studio, manning the phones and talking among themselves, and continually coming to me for direction and guidance, was somehow a bit too much for me. After an hour of that, I was starting to get really frazzled. My head was pounding, I felt a tightness in my chest, and my neck and shoulders felt like one of those knotted elastics that drive the propeller on a toy airplane. There was too much going on at once for me; I had become overstimulated. As a result, my effectiveness was seriously compromised, and everyone around me could see it. I could see the concerned looks on my friends' faces.

At that time, I was a meditator, but a wishy-washy one. For a week or so, I'd meditate every day and I'd feel great. But then I'd get busy or distracted or lazy, and blow it off. Even so, I knew that no matter how stressed out I became, or how long I'd let that meditation faculty lie fallow, a deep meditation of thirty minutes or so would unwind me and get me back on an even keel. I had studied meditation with several Eastern teachers, and once I had settled on some simple techniques that worked for me, I had found it a very wonderful tool for creating a more tranquil mind and a more peaceful life. Even so, my practice was not consistent. It was more what I'd call opportunistic—I meditated only when I felt the need.

Right then, I felt the need. My agitated state was compromising my effectiveness and threatening to undermine the whole project. However, with respect to the work at hand, there was no time to lose, and so, no time to meditate. My team of friends was available for that day only, we had a lot to accomplish, and we had just begun our work. Furthermore, I was the project leader; to absent myself for half an hour or more would have brought the whole project to a standstill.

I decided that as a palliative measure, a kind of psychological first aid, I would try a brief meditation of five minutes only. I didn't expect it to bring me all the benefits of that deep, half-hour plunge into stillness, but five minutes was all I felt I could spare. I hoped that those five minutes would at least blunt the edge of my distress so I could keep my team moving forward and function well enough to finish the job at hand.

Excusing myself, I went into the next room, closed the door, and settled myself on the simple chair that was my usual meditation perch. On any other day I would have joined my hands in the traditional way, palms up, left hand over right, tips of the thumbs touching. But this time, I did something different. For a few nights, I had been playing around with a new sleep technique. I don't remember how I got started on this, but I had taken to joining my hands in a curious way. Lying in bed, I would cross my thumbs and grasp my right thumb with the fingers of my left hand, and my left thumb with the fingers of my right. Then, each time I breathed in I would gently bend my wrists a little bit back, so my knuckles lifted up. Each time I breathed out, I'd relax. After several repetitions, I'd rest quietly, savoring the effect. I'd repeat that procedure as desired. This technique, which I called "the Healer," seemed very promising—after five or six rounds of it I'd enter a profoundly tranquil, sleeplike reverie. (I was later to learn from my colleague Josh Schreiber that this hand posture is offered in the Talmud as a remedy against demons who might otherwise get the upper hand when one has drunk unwisely: "And if a man forgot himself and happened to go out, what is his remedy? Let him take his right-hand thumb in his left hand and his left-hand thumb in his right hand . . .") Two updated versions of this technique, using a more comfortable hand posture, are included in chapter 4 in the sections "Main Squeeze" and "A Twist of the Wrists."

I had never really used the Healer during waking hours, however. After all, I was looking for bedtime sleep techniques, not daytime meditation techniques. Besides, I was perfectly happy with the traditional meditation techniques I already knew. They worked just fine, as far as I was concerned. However, since this was not to be a traditional half-hour meditation session, it seemed natural to try a nontraditional technique. I decided to try the Healer. I grasped my thumbs, lowered them to my lap, and closed my eyes. I focused my awareness on my breath, allowing it to become light, easy, slow, and soft. These qualities of breath, I had learned, provide a gradual, reliable entrée to deep meditation. At the same time, I became aware of very distinct feelings in my thumbs. They felt pleasantly warm, blanketed as they were by the fingers of the opposite hand. But more than that, I could feel a pulsation there, as well as a faint, pleasant, tingling sensation. I focused my attention on that sensation. Then I did a few rounds of movement, synchronizing the bending of my wrists with the gentle in-and-out flow of my breath, resting quietly for a time after each round. Soon enough, I had reached that same deeply restful state I'd achieved when I'd done the Healer in bed.

This restful state was not unlike the experiences I'd had in traditional meditation, but it seemed somehow deeper, easier, and more pleasurable. In meditation, I had always been trying to *achieve* something, even if that something was emptiness, or no-mind. Here, there was no effort, no striving of any kind. I was simply enjoying the experience of being myself, without any special goal or purpose. Instead of *doing*, I could simply *be*. For that moment, I was at peace, and I felt a deep sense of gratitude.

Then my five minutes were up, and it was time to go back to work. Back in the other room, my friends were still chugging along, getting their assigned jobs done, but I was a changed man. "What happened to you?" asked Julie. She could see and hear the difference in me immediately. My dark, tightly pinched face had cleared completely and my voice was an octave lower. My formerly grim expression was replaced by one of contentment. "And your eyes," she said, "they're twinkling!" The others agreed. I gave no explanation, but just smiled faintly. I wasn't even sure if what I had experienced was real. We all went back to work, and we were making good progress. Instead of feeling oppressed by the flurry of activity all around me, I was now relishing it. Where there had been strain and worry, there was now peace. Where there had been anxiety and effort, there was now ease. How different things seemed after that brief period of refreshment!

At one o'clock, we had a nice lunch together at a nearby restaurant, and we were back at work by two-fifteen. At three-thirty, I found myself slipping back into that tense, agitated state I'd encountered in the morning. At first I didn't notice it, but after a while somebody got a look at me and asked, "Are you all right?" That was a word to the wise, and besides, I was eager to repeat that easy, pleasurable, invigorating experience I'd had in the morning. Again I excused myself and went in the other room. Five minutes of the Healer, and I was myself again. By the time that special day drew to its fruitful conclusion, I had a delightful feeling of satisfaction. Wow, I thought to myself—this is great stuff! I've found a quick, efficient way to manage the stress of life, and it feels so good that I want to do it again and again.

I was so excited about this new technique and so curious about its potential effects that I decided to replace my occasional, half-hour meditation practice with brief, regular practice of the Healer. I wanted to see what the Healer could do if I really stuck to it. I started to practice two or three times a day, sometimes sticking to my five-minute limit, sometimes extending those periods of delicious repose to ten minutes. There was no real schedule. I'd do it at many different times: first thing in the morning, before lunch, in the late afternoon, at the end of the workday, in the late evening, or just before bed. With this modest, informal, but consistent practice I was experiencing really spectacular results. When I was hurried, the Healer helped me to slow down. When I was worried, the Healer helped me to stay focused on the moment. When I was harried, the Healer helped me to connect to an inner source of stability. This simple "movement meditation" technique, it seemed to me, had the power to reverse the effects of stress throughout the course of the day. I began to rely on the Healer as my day-to-day, moment-to-moment antidote to the stress of life.

I was to find that the Healer, and several other "movement meditation" techniques that I was to discover, were more than just a psychological first aid to apply every time life got to be too much for me. Gradually I came to understand that the Healer's effects were cumulative: The more I practiced, the calmer, steadier, and more stable my mind became. Those three, five-minute breaks in the action seemed to interrupt the vicious cycle of overstimulation and hyperarousal, allowing my nervous system to recalibrate itself to a slower, more natural rhythm of life and work. I was still leading the same life, doing the same work, living in the same city, but life was getting easier and more enjoyable. Life was getting more *peaceful*. Sure, I still had some nervous, anxious moments. I still got hurried, worried, and harried. But the peaks of nervousness, anxiety, and overstimulation were not as jagged; the valleys were neither so deep, nor so deeply shadowed. And that made a very big difference in the quality of my life.

Secrets of Sounder Sleep

This was a very fertile time for me. By day, in addition to my rewarding work as a Feldenkrais teacher, I was savoring the pleasure and the peace brought to me by those three brief episodes of movement meditation spread out over the course of the day. By night, I was developing new Mini-Moves to help myself deeply rest and sleep. Remember, falling asleep at bedtime had never been my problem; it was the prolonged periods of wakefulness later in the night that had given me trouble. Even so, at bedtime I would often lull myself to sleep with a Mini-Move, simply because I found this the easiest, most pleasurable way to drift off to sleep. I loved the way the Mini-Moves would ease me into sleep gradually. Then, if I happened to awaken some hours later, I'd do that same Mini-Move again and I'd be back asleep in a very short time. The periods of quiet rest following the gentle, synchronized movements and breathing would merge imperceptibly into hours of deep sleep. Even on my most challenging nights, when I might experience two or three awakenings, I was able to recover quickly each time. In that way, I'd string together several fragments of sleep, like the pearls on a necklace, into a single, virtually continuous night of natural sleep. Maybe those weren't my most restful nights ever, but they were restful nonetheless. On balance, I was getting more of the rest I needed, and life was sweeter and more livable as a result. I began to feel that, for myself at least, I had discovered the insomnia solution.

Synergy

It took me a little while to realize that these parallel processes, the Healer and other movement meditations by day and Mini-Moves by night, were working together in a synergistic manner. As I looked back over the preceding months, it became clear that the Mini-Moves had begun to produce their most marked sleep-inducing effects only after I'd started practicing the Healer in earnest. There must be a connection, I reasoned. By making my days more peaceful, my movement meditation practice was setting the scene for sounder sleep. As a result, I'd arrive at bedtime in just the right frame of mind and body for a night of natural, restful sleep. And by approaching bedtime in the right frame of mind and body, I'd seen how the sleep-inducing Mini-Moves I'd created had become all the more effective.

This conclusion was amply supported by my own experience and observation, but I would soon receive scientific confirmation of it as well. A 2001 study conducted at the Sleep Research and Treatment Center in the Department of Psychiatry at Pennsylvania State University reported that among a group of eleven young insomniacs who spent four nights in a sleep lab, there were increased plasma levels of the hormones cortisol and ACTH not only at bedtime, but twenty-four hours a day. The degree of hormonal elevation correlated positively with the degree of objective sleep disturbance—higher cortisol and ACTH meant worse sleep. Furthermore, these elevated hormonal secretions rose and fell in the same daily circadian rhythm as they do in normal sleepers.

Cortisol and ACTH are adrenal hormones produced by the hypothalamic-pituitary-adrenal (HPA) axis, which is your body's central control mechanism for the stress response. You can't do without these hormones; they play an essential role in maintaining arousal, and hence normal, waking consciousness throughout the day. And in an emergency, when you're under threat, attack, or duress—or when you believe that you are or merely suspect that you might be—they provide the quick energy you need to respond effectively to a dangerous situation. Your heart beats faster, your blood pressure is elevated, your muscle tone increases, your body temperature rises, and you break into a sweat, to name just a few of the typical physiological effects. When the threat passes, the hormones gradually subside, and your body returns to its regular, restful state. This is just as it should be.

But when you produce too much of these hormones, for too long, there's the devil to pay. Now, your heart beats consistently faster than normal, your blood pressure remains elevated, your muscles never fully relax, your body temperature is higher, and you sweat more all the time. In other words, your metabolism is elevated, and your whole system is working harder than it should. This is called physiological *hyperarousal*. That's what gives you that frazzled, over-the-edge feeling that comes with endless hurry, worry, and hassle during waking hours. And at night, when the two hormones ought to be at their lowest point, those same physiological effects can keep you up past your bedtime and produce shallow, fragmented, restless sleep and frequent awakenings.

These findings, the authors assert, indicate that insomnia is caused by chronic over-activation of the HPA axis, and is a disorder of "central nervous system hyperarousal" rather than a disturbance of the body's sleep-wake system. That could be bad news for insomniacs, they say, because it suggests that they may be at risk not only for mental disorders like anxiety and depression, but also for a host of stress-related illnesses. "The therapeutic goal in insomnia," they conclude, "should be to decrease the overall level of physiologic and emotional arousal, and not just to improve the nighttime sleep."

Gee whiz, I couldn't have said it better myself! Through my own experience and observation, I had discovered much the same thing that was described in the Pennsylvania State research. By day, movement meditation kept me cool, calm, and collected—so I could remain fully awake and engaged in my daily activities, but without becoming overstimulated, without crossing the line into frazzle. By night, I could use sleep-inducing Mini-Moves to create the internal mental and physical environment most conducive to easy, natural sleep. Working in tandem, the two techniques reduced my "overall level of physiologic and emotional arousal" by making my life more balanced and more peaceful, so I could get all the natural restful sleep I needed.

A "Sleep Soiree"

At the time I was making these discoveries, I used to teach two weekly Feldenkrais classes in my studio. The classes were not large, and the students were mostly folks I'd seen on a regular basis for months, and in some cases years. We knew each other well. The atmosphere was relaxed and informal, and the theme of the classes was adjusted from week to week according to the students' personal needs. When Ruth's back was sore from carrying her two-year-old, we explored a series of movements calculated to encourage her swift recovery. When Ron was singing an opera role in which he needed to fall down dead, we explored several different ways of falling down, and getting up again, with ease. When Joe was having trouble playing tennis without triggering an old shoulder injury, we did some lessons to address that challenge. And so on. Since Awareness Through Movement (ATM) classes address universal movement themes, and not specific ailments, everyone enjoyed the benefits of these classes, and we had a lot of fun in the bargain.

A quick poll of these old friends confirmed that there was sufficient interest to transform one of the classes into an experimental workshop for rest and sleep. I called it a "sleep soiree." "Oh boy," said Jan, an editor for a national magazine, "Do I ever need that!" We began meeting in the early evening every Tuesday night. Since this was something distinctly different in form and content from the classical Feldenkrais lessons I'd been teaching, I felt empowered to do things in my own personal way. I felt a deep gratitude and love for the Mini-Moves, and I wanted those feelings to be expressed in the way I taught. Also, most people would be coming directly from their jobs, so I wanted to begin with something that would undercut the tension of the workplace and create a mood of tranquility, contentment, and peace.

I began each class with soft, rhythmic Indian or Middle Eastern music. Sitting on mats on the floor or on stools, we did a series of gentle rocking and swaying movements inspired by Adnan Sarhan, the Sufi meditation teacher I had met a year earlier. The sweet music, the sensuous rhythms, and the lulling movements had a way of banishing all cares and rendering us receptive to deep rest and relaxation. After that musical interlude, I'd invite everyone to lie down on a mat on the floor and rest quietly. I'd turn down the lights, put on some very quiet flute music, and let everybody rest quietly for ten or fifteen minutes under my watchful eye. Some remained lucid during this initial nap period, others drifted off.

The rest period lasted about ten minutes. When it was over, I gently roused everyone and asked them to slowly sit up. I could see that the slow movements and the brief rest had produced the desired effect. The masks were down; everyone seemed more relaxed, open, and receptive to learning. I demonstrated the basic hand posture for the Healer and made sure everyone could do it on their own. Then I guided the group through two ten-minute movement meditations with a short break in between.

The result was very gratifying. Everyone was able to follow my simple instructions and they each arrived very quickly at a place of profound stillness and tranquility. Some expressed surprise at the result. Julie, a database manager whose natural sleep rhythms had been disturbed by years of night shift work, said that what we had done reminded her of meditation classes she had once attended. "But in the meditation class we were asked to focus on our breath," she explained, "and my mind just wandered all over the place. It took me forever to get settled." With the Healer she found it much easier to focus her attention on the movements synchronized with breathing, becoming deeply absorbed. Frederick said that he had experienced a profound sense of "letting go" of all cares. "It was a big relief," he said, smiling sheepishly. I turned to Jan, expecting some sort of comment from the usually voluble editor. For the moment speech, that "flimsiest of human faculties," had deserted her and she merely smiled and nodded her head slowly in appreciation. We all understood.

After the Healer, everyone lay down again and I guided the group in Breath Surfing, that first sleep-inducing Mini-Move that had delivered me from the grip of insomnia. They learned the basics, step by step, as well as a few variations I had devised along the way. Then I asked each person to choose the variation that gave them the most enjoyment, and to practice it on their own. It was fascinating to see with my eyes what I had previously only felt in my own body, and based on what I saw I made mental notes of things to experiment with on my own. Every seasoned teacher knows that they are likely to learn as much from their students as their students learn from them. This was no different.

There were five people in that first sleep soiree. After ten or so minutes of Breath Surfing, they had all fallen asleep. It was wonderful to see how quickly these hardworking folks, some of them confirmed insomniacs, could fall asleep given the right conditions! Laura, a hard-driving public relations exec, would later confess that this was the first time she'd fallen asleep without a sleeping pill in three years.

From the very first of these classes I loved watching people sleep. Most of us have had the experience of attending to a sleeping child. It's a pleasure to observe the soft, regular breathing, the blissful facial expressions, and all the little moves and murmurs children make during their descent into slumber. It's a pleasure also to sit by the bedside and savor the limpid silence and the air of innocence and goodwill that seem to emanate from the sleeping child. Well, I've discovered that adults are no different, just bigger! And here I had a room full of them, sleeping at my feet. It was delightful.

Frederick was a powerfully built, bearded psychologist well over six feet tall who, while awake, bore the fearsome expression of a biblical patriarch. But as he began to drift toward sleep, his elongated frame would curl up into a ball and his face, framed by the crook of one arm, would soften little by little until it assumed the expression of a very impish-looking little boy. Ellen, a former dancer turned real estate agent, had always had deeply etched vertical furrows between her eyebrows, as if she were endlessly puzzling over some complex mortgage formula. But now, as she hovered between waking and sleep, the dark furrows seemed to evaporate, and her smooth, oval face shone like translucent marble.

And it wasn't just Frederick and Ellen. It seemed to me that each person in the class had undergone a similar transformation as they passed from waking to sleep. It was as if each of them wore a mask displaying the image of themselves they wished to project to the world. In sleep the mask was miraculously lifted, revealing a softer, sweeter visage. In my view, this is a revelation of the person's original, unspoiled self, unencumbered by the stresses and strains of daily life. The physician and philosopher Sir Thomas Browne (1605–1682) seems to have shared this perception when he wrote: "We are somewhat more ourselves in our sleeps; and the slumber of the body seems to be the waking of the soul."

My subsequent experience has only reinforced this conviction.

For me, sleep is not only a biological process necessary for human life, but also a mechanism of the human spirit. That kernel of the true self, with its abundance of childlike goodness and generosity, slumbers within each one of us, no matter who we are or what we do. As we sleep, it works on us, rebuilding our vitality, lifting our spirits, and restoring our reserves of creativity, patience, and fellow-feeling. The proof? Just go without sleep for a couple of nights, and see what you become.

I let the nap go on for fifteen minutes or more. I put on a piece of rhythmic music, starting with the volume at zero and gradually bringing it up until it was just barely audible, enough to nudge people toward waking. Folks started to stretch and yawn. Our very first sleep soiree had reached its natural conclusion.

Word Spreads

Over the next weeks and months, I became a very eager proselytizer for the Mini-Moves. I wanted to share what I had discovered with as many people as possible. At the time I was seeing twenty or twenty-five clients a week for hour-long, individual Feldenkrais sessions. I began to ask everyone who came into my studio the simple question, "How do you sleep?" The result was startling. I found that unbeknownst to me, more than half of my clients were troubled sleepers. Some had intermittent bouts of sleeplessness, others had more frequent ones. Some simply didn't have enough *time* to sleep—extended work hours, long commutes, or family obligations had crowded sleep out of their weekly calendars, and onto the lower reaches of their to-do lists. At least among this small sampling of people, the sleep situation was far more dire than I had suspected. Within a few weeks, I was devoting about half my practice to sleep issues, with gratifying results. Word was getting around, and I was starting to get calls from clients' friends and family, who had heard about the Mini-Moves and wanted to try them for themselves. I was also teaching "Healing Sleep" classes at a senior citizens' center, and guest-speaking at a couple of NYPD precincts, teaching the Mini-Moves to patrol officers in full police gear, just before they hit the streets. It was really great to have so many opportunities to share my discoveries with so many people. The need was so acute.

I had begun to offer a second sleep soiree on Saturday mornings, and two of the regulars were a physical therapist, Fran, who was training to be a Feldenkrais teacher, and her mother. Mom had arthritis and couldn't get down to the floor, so I used to set up my padded Feldenkrais table for her in one corner of the room, and she'd lie there and follow all the movements as well as anyone. She was my biggest fan! Anyway, Fran began to lobby me about training her to teach the Mini-Moves. She wanted to offer a class to some of her patients in Westchester County. I was flattered, but I was really immersed in my own classes and private sessions, and the idea of training other professionals hadn't occurred to me. Fran's logic was convincing, however. She explained that by training other healing arts practitioners in the Mini-Moves, I could disseminate the Mini-Moves far more widely. Each health professional I trained would teach the Mini-Moves to many, many others. I began to think about starting a training group.

Teachers in Training

Our first professional training in the Sounder Sleep System began in January 2001. From among my Feldenkrais colleagues in the New York area I attracted a small but enthusiastic group of participants, including Jae Gruenke, Tyr Throne, John Copley Quinn, and Alta Ann Parkins Morris. We agreed to meet on Sundays, once a month, for a year. Feldenkrais teachers undergo an extensive process of experiential training that enables them to develop a very high level of sensitivity and self-awareness. They are experts at identifying those small differences in the way we think, act, and express ourselves that often make such a big difference in the quality of our lives. That made them a great sounding board for all the different techniques I'd developed. Together, we could discuss the best way to present this or that technique. We could talk about pacing, sequencing, the use of voice, and other technical issues. It was very enjoyable working closely with my colleagues in that small group, and we made many wonderful discoveries together.

I am very proud to report that all four of these early co-conspirators of mine went on to successfully teach the Mini-Moves in various settings. Jae has worked very effectively for SHARE, a support group for ovarian cancer survivors, through the community outreach programs of the New York Open Center, and in private practice. Tyr has taught sleep programs in Germany and Italy, and includes a Sounder Sleep module in the professional training program for his own Body Evolution method, which is an amalgam of rolfing, Feldenkrais, NLP (neuro-linguistic programming), yoga, and other somatic modalities. Alta Ann teaches napping workshops at Feldenkrais Associates, located high above New York's Union Square. And since September 11, 2001, my old friend John has served the city's beleaguered firemen and cops with utter selflessness—not a few times with the ruins of the World Trade Center still smoldering on their boots. Thank you, Jae, Tyr, Alta

"[The Mini-Moves] allow my system to heal itself, without imposing anything. Hooray!"

—STEVE SANDBERG,
musician and composer

Ann, and John, for your priceless contributions to the development and maturation of this work! I could see that training my colleagues in the Sounder Sleep System was going to be a very powerful way to deliver the Mini-Moves to the widest possible audience, as well as a richly rewarding experience in itself.

In May of that year, I began planning another training course in Los Angeles at the invitation of Dilys Tosteson Garcia and Avri Glick of Internal Ergonomics. I did not anticipate the many profound revelations I would experience as a result of this program. Our L.A. programs were held at the Beverly Hills studio of Claire Nettle, Feldenkrais teacher and trapeze artist extraordinaire— quite a switch from the Sounder Sleep System's gritty, overcast origins in Manhattan. I knew I had truly arrived in La-La-Land when Don Johnson of *Miami Vice* nearly bowled me over on his way out of the Starbucks on North Beverly Drive, and Lisa Kudrow of *Friends* jammed on the brakes of her SUV, graciously allowing me safe passage across Santa Monica Boulevard. I just love the way vehicles stop for pedestrians in California. In New York, it's the other way round!

Healing Sleep

Our New York training program met on twelve Sundays spread out over a year, but I couldn't possibly do that in Los Angeles. So we decided on a three-part format, meeting for three days each time. I would fly to Los Angeles in August, December, and April, and in that way we'd complete a slightly pared-down version of the New York program. It was a purely practical decision, but one that was to have the wonderful outcome of revealing to me the principle of Healing Sleep. Here's the background.

In Los Angeles we met for three days at a time, Friday through Sunday, starting at 10 a.m. and finishing at 5 p.m. Our group included twenty-three people from a variety of professions—nurses, physical therapists, Feldenkrais teachers and other movement educators, an acupuncturist, a school teacher, and others. And let me assure you that in spite of all those professional credentials, there were just as many troubled sleepers among this group as you would find in any group of your neighbors. Therefore, the purpose of our gathering was not only to train teachers, but also to help the troubled sleepers among them just as I had done with my clients in New York. That was fine with me, because I wanted my students to see me teaching the Sounder Sleep System in a real-life setting.

The daily schedule typically went something like this: We'd start the day with soothing, rhythmic instrumental music and some of those slow rocking and swaying movements I'd used in the original sleep soirees, which I had come to call "sleep yoga." Then we'd rest quietly for ten or twenty minutes. Next we'd have forty-five minutes or so of "guided natural breathing"—effortless breathing techniques designed to restore the natural rhythm and shape of the breath, which is often the first casualty of the pace of modern life. (L.E.S.S. Is More and Making Room in chapter 4 are examples of this class of techniques.) By now the room would be very peaceful. People would be deeply relaxed, perhaps drifting in and out of sleep, perhaps in a state of lucid, waking rest. Then, after a break, we'd all take chairs and practice some variation of the Healer, Main Squeeze, or a Twist of the Wrists (the latter two are also in chapter 4), culminating in fifteen or twenty minutes of silent meditation. After another short break, I'd take questions or comments, maybe give a short talk, and then we'd break for lunch.

In the afternoon, I might ask everyone to take a partner for some hands-on sleep-induction techniques. Technique is actually the wrong word, because these were more like experiments in perception and consciousness than fixed techniques. For example, in one of these experiments the resting partner would lie down, and the active partner would sit at her side, holding one of her hands. The active partner would place his thumb gently in the center of the resting partner's palm, and with that thumb he'd very slowly and gradually stretch the skin of the palm a little bit this way, a little bit that way, finally culminating in small, slow circles. The resting partner's job was to just lie quietly, and feel the effect of those minimal movements on her mood and her state of attention and arousal. This is wonderful stuff—the person touches only your hand, but gradually every part of you is suffused with a feeling of profound well-being. And if you need sleep, you will almost certainly fall into a state of peaceful slumber. After twenty minutes of that, the two partners would briefly exchange observations and switch roles. Next I might introduce a longer sequence of Lulling Mini-Moves, lying first on the back, then on the side, and perhaps on the belly. People invariably wander in and out of sleep during these teachings. That is, they learn the Mini-Moves by actually putting them into practice. After an hour or more of that, everyone would be in a state of profound repose, including me, so I'd put on some soothing music at a barely audible volume and let everyone rest for an extended period. Then, as the day drew to a close, I'd take a few more questions or give a lecture on some sleep-related topic. Then we'd break for the day.

As you can see, this is not your average professional training program in the healing arts. First of all, there is a much greater emphasis on actually experiencing the Mini-Moves than on learning facts or theories. Medically or scientifically oriented courses rarely afford students the time to stop and actually feel the physical sensations associated with any of the things they are learning; the emphasis is on cramming facts into the limited space of the student's cranium. But this is most assuredly not a medically oriented course, and that fact- and theory-oriented model of learning is not at all appropriate for the Mini-Moves. To teach the Mini-Moves, you have to know them deep down in your bones, in your body and soul. It's not enough to just know the sequence of movements, like the points on an academic syllabus. Rather, you learn to completely recalibrate your senses to a much slower, more subtle level, so you can actually feel the gradual process that unfolds inside you, not only in your muscles and nerves, but also in your mind, as you fall asleep. Once you are attuned in that way, the Mini-Moves become an intrinsic part of you. Then, not only do you get the maximum benefit from practicing them yourself, but also you are able to communicate them to others most effectively.

It's ironic, but I myself have never had the experience of attending one of these rather extraordinary gatherings, except as the teacher. And as the teacher I have to be wide awake the whole time—I don't get to lie down and have someone guide me through five or six hours of Mini-Moves a day for three days running. Therefore, the experiences that my students have, and the many, many discoveries that they have made as they explore their inner landscape during these extended programs, are always a real revelation for me. Here are a few examples:

Suze Angel, a single mom from Laguna Beach who teaches the Feldenkrais Method, qigong, and other movement arts to adults and seniors all over Orange County, wrote: "Since my early twenties I have suffered from periodic insomnia, waking up in the middle of the night with a racing mind and not being able to go back to sleep. During the Sounder Sleep™ workshop I had so many wonderful, refreshing naps. Following the workshop, my abdomen and breathing are more profoundly relaxed than they have been since the birth by Caesarean section of my son nine years ago, and I am finally caught up on my sleep. Thank you for the best rest I can remember!"

Peter Hasson, who leads a triple life as a psychotherapist, an international tour organizer, and an extremely talented painter, had joined the workshop to pick up a few extra skills to use with his clients. But he promptly found a warm place for the Mini-Moves in his own heart. "I came away with the profound knowledge of how to calm myself down and to find my own center," Peter reports. "Now, I can focus better and deal with the stress of each day by practicing the Mini-Moves. The Sounder Sleep System is so easy to learn, and it really works." And naturally, Peter has shared these same profound skills with many of his clients, as well.

Jean Ashby is a businesswoman from Newport Beach who suffers from sleep apnea, a condition in which breathing stops at intervals during the night. She gave the following account of her experience with the workshops: "Since I learned the Sounder Sleep System I get more rest from the hours I spend in bed, so I'm sleeping more efficiently. Getting the sleep I need is more pleasurable and less work. I've experienced a significant reduction in anxiety, so I'm calmer and more at ease by night and day."

"I used to fight to stay awake during the day," Jean continues, "but I didn't know I was doing it. Now I'm much more aware of my own sleepiness, and I feel no qualms about napping as needed. But my naps are much more efficient: fifteen minutes usually does the trick, instead of three hours. All in all, I have achieved a much greater degree of self-acceptance." Please note that the Mini-Moves are not a cure for apnea. Jean still relies on her continuous positive airway pressure (CPAP) machine, which maintains positive airway pressure throughout the night. But isn't it nice to know that the Mini-Moves can make life with sleep apnea easier and more enjoyable?

Yet another of these revelations was first articulated by Dilys Garcia. Dilys was one of those people who really resists sleep. She told us that she has always been inclined to put sleep off as long as possible, thinking that there were so many more interesting things she'd rather do. As a result, she was accustomed to staying up late, sleeping only a few hours a night, and starting her day early in the morning. Yet throughout these first three L.A. gatherings, Dilys repeatedly expressed surprise at how very deeply, and how long, she slept on the nights of the training. As it turned out, many of the other students had this same experience, and we were quite surprised by it at first. After all, one of the key mechanisms determining our sleep-wake rhythm is the *sleep homeostat*. It works like this: The longer you've been awake, the stronger will be the drive to sleep, and conversely, the longer you sleep, the less inclined you'll be to sleep. That's one reason why you tend to feel very sleepy late at night, after being awake all day, and fully alert when you awaken after a good night's sleep. Now if you spent the whole day meandering in and out of sleep as the participants in these programs did, you might think that you wouldn't be inclined to sleep much on the following nights. All that resting, dozing, and dreaming during the daytime ought to have turned down the sleep homeostat, reducing your sleep drive considerably. But it seems that just the opposite is true, according to the reports of many people who have attended my programs, not only in those first Beverly Hills gatherings, but all over the world in the years that followed. In many cases, those days spent lying down and deeply, truly resting make it possible to go home and sleep more deeply than you ever did before. And the effect is most pronounced following the third day. And best of all, when the program's over that effect can be sustained indefinitely by regular home practice of the Mini-Moves. Based on this experience, we have come to the conclusion that *we sleep deepest and most restfully not when we're totally exhausted or fatigued, but when we are deeply, truly, relaxed.* This is the principle of Healing Sleep.

"As a maternity nurse, I've found these techniques to be great for calming patients' anxiety. For myself, I always do them lying down because I am certain to fall sleep within minutes!"
— CALLY PHELAN, *RN*

Another fascinating observation we made during these three-day programs was that when you give people the opportunity to deeply rest for three days at a time, they soak it up like a sponge! Nowadays we spend so much of our time in feverish activity that we assume that activity is our natural state. We go, go, go all day long and then sleep for six or seven or eight hours in order to recover and restore our vital energies. Then we wake up and do it all over again, assuming that we've had all the rest our bodies need. Yet here was a group of two dozen thoughtful, busy, creative professionals who, given the opportunity, could happily remain in a state of quiet rest, meditation, introspection, contemplation, or sleep for three days at a stretch. And not only did they enjoy it enormously and feel more relaxed, alert, and alive afterward, but they also could go home at the end of the day to sleep through the night.

That really started me thinking about the issue of how much rest and sleep people truly need. And I realized that there is a huge gulf between the minimum amount of rest we *need* and the maximum amount of rest we can *use*. We *need* seven, eight, or nine hours of sleep, or whatever it takes just to get each of us through the day. That's purely a matter of survival. But we can *use* a whole lot more. We can use more sleep, and we can use more time to rest, contemplate, imagine, and dream. We can use more time in which to cease *doing*, and simply *be*. When we get a healthy dose of that kind of rest, something shifts inside of us. In physiological terms, we can assume that there is a shift away from the dominance of the sympathetic branch of the autonomic nervous system, which triggers arousal and the stress response, and a shift toward dominance of the parasympathetic branch, which triggers our resting and recuperative faculties. We go from the energy-intensive "fight or flight" mode to energy-conserving, "rest and digest" mode, and we stay there, relaxing and recuperating, drifting in and out between waking and sleep, for a prolonged period of time. The more of that we do, the more our minds and bodies slow down, our hearts open up, and we develop a more gracious relationship with time. As a result, we are more at ease, both physically and mentally, we feel better, look better, and enjoy life more.

With this in mind, it's interesting to note the results of a recent study of sleep extension conducted at Stanford University under the supervision of William C. Dement, the godfather of American sleep research. A group of fifteen healthy college students reporting minimal daytime sleepiness were monitored for five nights during which they maintained their normal sleep schedules, then were allowed to sleep as much as possible during two sleep extension periods, one lasting seven days, and another immediately following it of six to forty-eight days. (Subjects left the experiment once they had reached maximum alertness levels and felt that they could no longer gain extra sleep, or when outside commitments required it.) The students were continuously monitored by means of a wrist actigraph, a wristwatch-like device that records sleep-wake activity; it recorded their bedtime, sleep latency (time it takes to fall asleep), rise time, naps, total hours slept, and a subjective rating of mood in daily journals.

What were the results? You guessed it. There was a considerable increase in sleep among all participants, as compared to the baseline period. The students' average sleep times, which hovered around eight hours per night during the baseline period, soared up to ten hours and more on the first three nights of the sleep extension period, and then gradually declined as their sleep homeostat approached the satiety point. And what's more, that period of extended sleep led to improvements in daytime alertness, physical reaction time, and mood that were both objectively measurable and subjectively felt. As you can see, these results are quite congruent with what we observed in our Beverly Hills encounters.

The Circle Widens

Upon completion of this series of presentations in Los Angeles, I saw clearly that my work was only just beginning. It had been clear for some time that the Mini-Moves had tremendous potential to help people to help themselves. I wanted to share that message with a broader public. To that end, I had trained two groups of teachers, one in New York and one in California, who would go on to share the Mini-Moves with far more people than I could do single-handedly. But in California, I had discovered something unexpected, which was that the Mini-Moves could produce even more potent effects when presented in an extended format that gave participants plenty of time to relax, rest, and recover while learning. There was something special about giving yourself three days to rest quietly in a state of profound repose, surrounded by others who did the same. And I believed that this would be just as true for the average person suffering from insomnia and the stress of life as it was for the practitioners I had trained. Thus the Healing Sleep retreat was conceived.

Over the next few years, we would begin opening our three-day gatherings to members of the general public as well as to the healing arts practitioners. We offered the same three-day format (sometimes offering a two-day option for those who couldn't spare three), and the same combination of the experiential and the didactic, but we offered it to a mixed group of practitioners and public. In programs in Seattle, Baltimore, New York, Chicago, and other cities and towns around the United States, we began to explore the possibilities of these Healing Sleep retreats, and we found that our non-practitioners fit in perfectly. The personal sleep-related challenges and concerns were a wonderful, vitalizing addition to our usual curriculum, and our usual manner of operating was slow enough and nurturing enough to accommodate just about anyone with a sincere interest in participating.

During that time, I would witness many examples of personal transformation that comes with three days of profound, thoroughgoing rest accompanied by the practice of Mini-Moves. For example, a woman I'll call Paula attended one of our programs in Baltimore. Paula arrived late, so I didn't get a chance to meet her beforehand. But I knew the moment I looked at Paula that there was quite a struggle going on inside of her. Her face was drawn and contracted, as if she had just swallowed something extremely bitter, and had a grayish cast. She seemed extremely restless and uncomfortable, even though she was well supplied with mats, pillows, blankets, and warm socks. A few times during that day, I noticed she had broken into quiet tears and then fallen into a fitful sleep. I kept my eye on Paula, making sure that she was able to follow the thread of my teaching and offering quiet encouragement for her successes in doing so. I made a mental note to speak with her privately to see if any special support was needed. But when I asked after her at the end of the day, I found that she had slipped out a little early to take care of some personal errands. By the second day she seemed more at ease, a little more peaceful. Again, she eluded my efforts to make contact. On the third morning of the program, Paula arrived with a huge smile on her face. She was positively radiant! "What happened to you?" I asked. "Last night I slept through the night for the first time in thirteen years," Paula explained. "I feel wonderful!"

We have heard similar reports from many other Healing Sleep attendees. A young lawyer named "Jane" attended a program I gave at the Kripalu Center for Yoga and Health, a former Jesuit retreat perched on the shores of a sylvan lake in the Berkshire mountains of Massachusetts. At the time of the program, Jane hadn't had a good night's sleep in over two months. The problem had started just before she took the bar exam. By the time she started a new job with a litigation firm the following week, Jane was really in trouble. She was so exhausted and so impaired from lack of sleep that she responded with terror each time she was given a new work responsibility. She feared she was not cut out to be a lawyer. During our Kripalu program, Jane slept a lot. I could see that she had a lot of catching up to do! Even so, she learned enough to practice on her own, and her practice quickly bore fruit. Following the program, Jane regained her natural sleep rhythm and was soon sleeping almost eight hours each night. Not only was Jane's law career saved, but she was really beginning to enjoy it. "Things have really improved dramatically since the Healing Sleep retreat," she wrote. "I am looking forward to my first trial with excitement!"

Today, I give about twenty-five Healing Sleep retreats each year in various cities in the United States and Europe. Like those first programs in Los Angeles, they are attended by both healing-arts practitioners and members of the general public. I always feel honored when, as is often the case, people come from great distances to attend my programs. I enjoy teaching, and I'm always very grateful for any opportunity to share what I know with an enthusiastic audience. Of course, for every person that can attend one of my programs in person, there are many, many more who would like to attend, but can't. That's why I am writing this book. It is my hope that this book will make these helpful and much-needed techniques available to a wider audience.

Chapter 2

★ ★ ★ ★

How to Use This Book

So now you know something about the Sounder Sleep System and the Mini-Moves. You know how and why they came into being, you know a little bit about how they are taught, and you know what kinds of results they produce. In this chapter, I'll tell you about this book and how to make the most of the instructional materials contained in it. That way, you'll enjoy much the same kind of guidance and supervision I provide for the participants in my live programs.

This book is about self-healing. It teaches you to use your own physical movements and breath to overcome insomnia and get all the natural, restful sleep you need. In the process, you will heal your relationship with sleep. That means that your feelings about sleep and your attitudes toward sleep will change. Instead of dreading bedtime as a time of irritation, uncertainty, or disappointment, you will look forward to it as a time of comfort, pleasure, and peace. That is my goal for you, dear reader, and I have done everything in my power to help you achieve it with the means you hold in your hands.

Learning the Mini-Moves

The Sounder Sleep System is the basis of the insomnia solution presented in this book. The system is primarily an *oral* teaching, taught through the medium of speech and language either in live presentation or on recordings. There is also a secondary visual component, because in a live setting the teacher may demonstrate certain movements, and illustrations are usually provided along with recorded programs. But the core experience of learning and practicing the Mini-Moves happens with eyes closed, while listening to spoken instructions from a teacher. After all, it is with our eyes closed that we are most likely to deeply relax and sleep.

One of the challenges of creating this book has been to translate this fundamentally oral teaching into an illustrated text format so that you can learn the basics of the Sounder Sleep System by means of verbal instructions and visual illustrations. Great care has been taken to make this not only possible but also easy and enjoyable. When you are first learning the Mini-Moves, you will need to read them from the book or have someone read them to you. Reading them for yourself can be a bit of a challenge: Each time you start to get relaxed, you'll have to spoil the mood by opening your eyes and picking up the book to find out what is the next step. Clearly, that would be an impediment to your learning and enjoyment of the Mini-Moves. Not insurmountable, but an impediment nonetheless.

For that reason, I'm going to suggest a few simple, practical strategies for learning the Mini-Moves in this book. One is that you ask a family member, friend, or neighbor to read them aloud for you. In that case, choose someone who will take the time to read slowly and clearly, pausing as needed to allow you time to savor the effects of each step. Ideally, they should read one step at a time and then wait for you to indicate your readiness to move on with a nonverbal cue of some sort, for example, a sigh, a whispered word of your choosing, or any other signal you can give without arousing yourself too much. I have tested this method, and it works quite nicely. The key is choosing a sympathetic reader who is committed to helping you learn. If you can find someone with whom to trade, so that you later take a turn reading the Mini-Moves to them, that is a very wonderful way to learn and share. This also makes it easier to remember the Mini-Moves, since you are bound to go through each Mini-Move at least twice, once as the listener, and once as the reader. The complementary action of those two approaches, listening and reading aloud, is quite a powerful aid to memory, in my experience.

Another wonderful way to learn is to form a Mini-Move study group. Here you would gather a group of three to five family members, friends, or neighbors, all of whom are eager to learn. One person reads a Mini-Move aloud, while the others listen and follow the instructions. Then, someone else takes a turn reading the same Mini-Move again, so that the first reader gets a chance to try it, too. Continue like that, until everyone has had a chance to practice each Mini-Move. And of course you will want to practice what you learned as much as possible between meetings, too, so you can report back to each other as you progress. The factor of group support is another powerful aid to learning, memory, and enjoyment. When one or more members of the group start to experience favorable results and report their experiences to the others, the effect is contagious. After a while, group members may start to feel sleepy the moment they arrive at the meeting, and that same effect can be carried over into their own bedrooms.

Another possibility is that you may wish to record the Mini-Moves in your own voice so you can listen whenever you like. You are welcome to record the Mini-Moves for your personal use.

When you record, be sure to read slowly and clearly, and allow a pause of several complete breath cycles after each step is complete. Naturally, you can always pause the recording should you need more time to explore a given movement. But it's best to try to establish a nice, slow, rhythmic pace with frequent, long pauses on the recording itself. That way you won't have to fumble with the controls while you're trying to relax and learn. Finally, you may wish to purchase prerecorded programs of the Mini-Moves from one of the sources listed in appendix A. And of course, you are welcome to attend one of our live programs. A list of upcoming programs is always available on our Web site at soundersleep .com.

Three Types of Mini-Moves: Relax, Calm, and Lull

As you know, the Mini-Moves are designed to relax your body, calm your mind, and lull you to sleep. In accordance with this principle, the Mini-Moves in this book are divided into three types: Relaxing Mini-Moves (chapter 3) to reduce muscular tension and help you move with greater ease and enjoyment; Calming Mini-Moves (chapter 4) to help you achieve a calm, clear mind and a more peaceful life; and Lulling Mini-Moves (chapter 5) to help you fall asleep at bedtime or recover from nighttime awakenings. You will find ample description, explanation, and instruction in all three kinds of Mini-Moves in the associated chapters, along with plenty of helpful tips and friendly encouragement. For now, all you need to know is that you will probably need to learn and master at least one or two Mini-Moves of each type, depending on your own individual needs. But how will you decide where to begin and how to go on from there? That's what we're going to talk about next.

Tense, Nervous, Sleepless: What's Your Type?

If you're reading this book, you are almost certainly a troubled sleeper, but what type of troubled sleeper are you? Let's talk about that, because it will be a good indicator of where you can most profitably begin your practice of the Mini-Moves. Please note that this simple typology is based on pedagogical principles and is not a medical diagnosis. It is just a convenient tool to help you decide how much emphasis to place on each of the three types of Mini-Moves as you embark on the path toward self-healing.

Tense?

Tom was *tense*. Tom was a musician and journalist in his late thirties. When we met, he was nursing a sore wrist he'd developed while playing blues guitar. He suffered from a recurring stiff neck that seemed to get worse whenever a deadline was looming on the horizon. His dentist had informed him that he was grinding his teeth and suggested an appliance to forestall any further damage to his enamel. Tom spoke quickly and decisively, in a kind of staccato rhythm, and expected others to do the same. When I paused to think in the middle of a sentence, he'd finish it for me.

And on top of all that, or more likely because of it, Tom couldn't sleep. He'd often stay up until 3 a.m. writing, catch three or four hours of fitful sleep, have breakfast, and then pace the streets of New York for a couple of hours with a cup of takeout coffee in his hand. (I happened to be downstairs when he arrived for his first session with me, and that first mental snapshot of him abides to this day.) Then he'd spend the rest of the day at his desk, typing, typing, typing, gulping coffee, and telephoning the occasional interview subject. By the way, he was one of those who like to cradle the phone in the crook of their shoulder. He got the headset lecture *and* the coffee lecture during our first meeting!

My first intervention with Tom was a series of movement-awareness lessons of the type you'll find in chapter 3. These were meant to help him let go of some of that excess muscular tension and learn to sit, type, and play the guitar with greater comfort, ease, and efficiency. We even worked on his walk, for his heel-pounding, over-striding walking style was really doing some violence to his body. I figured that until we got some of that physical tension out of the way, there wasn't likely to be much improvement in his sleep behavior. Even though we associate it primarily with daytime activities, excess muscular tension can overflow into your bedroom, delaying the onset of sleep and giving it a shallow, fragmented quality.

Light, easy movement was a quite unfamiliar concept at first, but Tom eventually came to understand its value. At the beginning of our fourth meeting, he laughingly said, "You know, since we started working together, I'm doing everything just a little more softly. I'm *pussyfootin'!*" That was quite an admission from this hardboiled native New Yorker! And sure enough, once Tom started pussyfootin', some of his neck and wrist problems began to abate, and he started finding it a little easier to surrender to the waves of bedtime sleepiness that would make landfall at around ten and that he had previously ignored. I was very pleased when he announced that one of his New Year's resolutions was to be in bed before midnight on at least five nights of the week. Can you guess what any of the others were? (Hint: headset, caffeine.)

At the same time, I began to introduce Tom to some of the Calming Mini-Moves, and we found one (Main Squeeze, chapter 4) that was particularly pleasing to him. He agreed to practice it twice a day, once before lunch and once in the late evening. Later, he told me he found it soothing to do it briefly during his breaks from writing, too—he didn't feel the need to drink so much coffee as a result. "I'm happier and more productive when I'm relaxed than when I'm in caffeine catastrophe mode," he averred. Of course, the reduced caffeine input had its effect, too. Less caffeine equals a lower arousal level, which makes sleep all the more possible and likely.

Tom became quite adept at the Calming Mini-Move we had chosen for him, and he was really enjoying its cumulative, tranquilizing effects. His voice seemed to have become softer and lower, and he no longer finished my sentences for me. As he left one of our sessions, I went down in the elevator with him to observe his departure. As he headed for Central Park, he was indeed pussyfootin'. That kinder, gentler walk was a pleasure to watch.

Tom was now at the point where I felt he was ready to practice some of the Lulling Mini-Moves (chapter 5). We tried a few different ones, and Tom liked the Ziggurat, so he started with that. He began, as I always insist, by *practicing during waking hours*, substituting a Lulling Mini-Move for one of his Main Squeeze breaks in the late afternoon. After several days of that, he could practice fluently without having to think too much about it, so I encouraged him to try the Ziggurat in bed, at bedtime only. Of course, falling asleep at bedtime was not Tom's problem—it was those late-night awakenings, as is true for the majority of troubled sleepers. But by Tom's doing the Mini-Move at bedtime, when he was most likely to fall asleep, we were gradually getting his mind and body habituated to the idea that when he did those movements, he was going to fall asleep. I utilize some variation of this principle of gradual implementation, which I call "the Waiting Game," with virtually all of my clients. And I recommend it to you, too. This won't be the last mention of it in this book!

The Waiting Game certainly worked for Tom, because some

days later, when I gave him the okay to use the Mini-Move in response to his early-morning awakenings, he found that this by-now very well practiced Mini-Move got him back to sleep in no time. As a result, this three-hour-a-night man was able to sleep from midnight to 6 a.m. He had doubled his sleep total! And that was just the beginning. In the weeks that followed, with some gentle prompting from me, Tom began going to bed at 11 or 11:30, waking up briefly at 3 a.m. for personal needs and a sip of water, and then, with the aid of the Ziggurat, sleeping soundly until 7 a.m. Tom was now sleeping seven and a half to eight hours a night, and loving it. He'd also begun to practice Breath Surfing, another of the Lulling Mini-Moves. He found that he valued the flexibility of being able to fall asleep on his back, too.

Does Tom's situation sound familiar? Do you suffer from excessive physical tension? Do you tend to grind your teeth, clench your fists, or stop your breathing? Do you get frequent backaches, stiff necks, tendinitis, eyestrain, or other nagging aches and pains? Do you find that ordinary everyday movements often require more flexibility or range of motion than you can muster? Do you walk with the force of a locomotive, twist faucets until the washers cry uncle, and pound the keys of your keyboard 'til they ring like a blacksmith's anvil? Maybe, whether you're aware of it or not, you're suffering from excess muscular tension. (Naturally, you'll want to consult your doctor to determine whether there are any medical causes behind these complaints.)

If you do suffer from excess tension, this may very well be one of the causes of your troubled sleep. In that case, I suggest you look carefully at the Relaxing Mini-Moves in chapter 3, and begin your practice there. Read the text, look at the pictures, see what attracts you. That will get you started on the road to greater lightness and ease of movement, to greater relaxation and reduced effort in your daily activities, with many of the same salutary effects that Tom experienced. Who knows, you may even find that, like Tom, you like yourself better this way! How often should you practice the Relaxing Mini-Moves? Whenever you can. Can you do one a week? That's great. Twice? Even better. The key is to really take the time to do them slowly and mindfully, without hurry. That will ensure that you get the best results.

At the same time, please take the time to master one or two of the Calming Mini-Moves in chapter 4 and, as Tom did, practice two or three times a day for ten minutes or more. You'll find that they, too, will make a valuable contribution to the quality of your life and work. Tense people almost invariably need both Relaxing and Calming Mini-Moves. Nervousness and anxiety seem to go hand in hand with excessive physical tension, and both can keep you awake. Finally, visit the Lulling Mini-Moves in chapter 5. They will put the icing on the cake, teaching you how to fall asleep at bedtime, and how to recover quickly if you wake up during the night. For further advice on how to most fruitfully develop your practice of the Calming and Lulling Mini-Moves, follow the Basic Program, below.

Nervous?

> To allow oneself to be carried away by a multitude of conflicting concerns; to surrender to too many demands; to commit oneself to too many projects; to want to help everyone in everything; is itself to succumb to the violence of our times.
> —THOMAS MERTON

Andrea was the nervous type. A former schoolteacher in her mid-sixties, she was retired in name only. She lived with two pampered cats in a pleasant, sunny private home filled with children's art and native crafts collected over the course of a lifetime. Even though she was no longer working for a living, Andrea's days were jam-packed with activities—charity work, environmental activism, and visits to all the local schools to share with the younger generation her lifelong fascination with ecology and conservation. As the recipient of several scholarly grants, she had become quite an expert on the subject. She found it all very rewarding, but after a full day like that, Andrea was losing sleep. She had no trouble falling asleep, but she'd wake up at three or four in the morning, unable to return to sleep.

There were some immediate physical causes for Andrea's sleeplessness—an irritable hip with possible arthritic involvement, a nagging digestive problem that wasn't responding to any of the prescribed remedies. Of course, these and any other medical issues were being addressed by Andrea with her medical providers. But when I met Andrea, the first thing that caught my attention was her nervousness, overstimulation, and hyperarousal. You see, Andrea was keeping busy in retirement, and that's good, but there was a driven quality to her busyness. She could go, she could do, but she could not stop, she could not just *be*. After each of our meetings, she would open her day planner to schedule our next appointment, and I would always marvel at how every time slot was filled. I've known successful doctors and lawyers whose schedule contained more wiggle room than Andrea's. Often, she would have to cancel something else in order to fit me in. Then, she'd call me the next day to see if we could meet fifteen minutes earlier, or a half hour later than we had agreed. She was shoehorning each new appointment into her already loaded schedule. In addition, Andrea was a bit of a perfectionist, highly conscientious in all her affairs and undertakings. That meant that she couldn't just do something and be done with it; she had to evaluate the outcome and figure out a better way to do it in the future. This, too, is a good quality, not a bad one. But when you consider the sheer volume of Andrea's activities and add to that the intensity of commitment she gave to each one, and add to that her troubled sleep, you start to suspect that something could be out of balance.

When I questioned Andrea about the causes of her sleeplessness, she mentioned the sore hip and the anguished gut, but she did not seem to be aware of the role played by her mind. But with closer questioning, she admitted that her habit of unceasing thought, planning, evaluation, and re-planning might be one of the factors keeping her awake. Upon reflection, she came to realize that her nocturnal awakenings were more often than not triggered by thoughts that seemed to bubble up out of the depths of sleep. Sometimes she would awaken from a sound sleep and bolt out of bed to write herself yet another reminder of something she must do the next day, or a new project she must undertake. Andrea aptly summarized the problem as follows: "It's not that I wake up, and then begin to think; it's that I begin to think, and those thoughts awaken me. I didn't think such a thing was possible."

It is possible, however. A study of thoughts and hallucinations in waking and sleep conducted at the University of Oslo, Norway, by Fosse, Stickgold, and Hobson, some of our most imaginative sleep researchers, indicates that our thinking diminishes only gradually throughout the first stages of sleep, finally reaching its nadir in the REM sleep phase, which is dominated instead by those very convincing, emotionally charged hallucinations we call dreams. I believe that Andrea was living proof of this finding. After an overly stimulating day of highly compressed activities, she would fall into a shallow sleep marked by relatively high levels of non-dreaming thought. In other words, she was still chewing on all those meaty thought processes that she'd initiated during the day but hadn't had time to digest. At a certain point, some particularly potent thought would impose itself on Andrea's awareness, heightening her already elevated arousal enough to wake her up. And then, the ensuing stream of thoughts and feelings would keep her aroused and awake for the rest of the night.

In light of this, I decided that one of the Calming Mini-Moves would be the best place for Andrea to begin her quest for sounder sleep. It would create some much needed time-outs in the course of her day, and at the same time reduce some of the cognitive overload that was keeping her in that nervous, restless, sleep-deprived state. We began with L.E.S.S. Is More, just as it is presented in chapter 4. Andrea took to that simple exercise right away, finding that it instantly brought her a feeling of peace and well-being that had long eluded her. We agreed that she would take two or three daily time-outs of ten minutes each in order to practice the technique.

My plan was to wait until Andrea had achieved considerable mastery of that first Relaxing Mini-Move, and perhaps one other, and had begun to enjoy some of the cumulative relaxing effects. As we were establishing this daily practice, I would begin to introduce the option of reducing her activity level ever so slightly, to leave more time for rest and reflection. I was eager to see some gaps in that day planner of hers! Only later, when Andrea was well settled in her practice, would we begin to experiment with some of the Lulling Mini-Moves, until we found the one or two that she could use most fruitfully when she awoke in the wee hours. That would be what I'd do with anyone who, like Andrea, was the nervous, overstimulated type.

Andrea surprised me, however. In the week following our meeting, she not only practiced that Mini-Move during those two or three daytime rest periods, but also during the night. She had discovered that, for her, it could be a very pleasurable and peaceful way to drift off to sleep at bedtime and also a powerful aid to recovering her sleep if she awoke during the night. She found that on the days when she stuck to her daytime practice regimen, her sleeping mind was far less active, far less likely to wake her up. A curious and welcome side effect was that Andrea's digestive problems had begun to abate during that same week. "Maybe the medicine's finally taking effect," she speculated. Maybe so. But the gut is one of those places that are particularly sensitive to the effects of stress. Reduce the stress, and the gut has a chance to recover. And that Mini-Move had certainly reduced Andrea's stress level.

In any case, Andrea was very happy with the results of our work together. She was sleeping longer and more deeply, and if she did awaken at any time during the night, she could get herself back to sleep within a reasonable time. Later, I did teach her some of the Lulling Mini-Moves, and she loved experimenting with the different effects that each one produced. Still, she maintained an abiding fondness for that first Calming Mini-Move she had learned, L.E.S.S. Is More. She practiced every day, and at night it was her favorite tool for recovering from those premature awakenings. Andrea and I continued meeting for several weeks more. We experimented with a variety of movements designed to relieve some of the stress on her hip in walking and sitting. When we last met, Andrea's hip was almost fully recovered, and all the signs of golden sleep were written on her smiling face.

Does Andrea's story ring a bell for you? Might you be the nervous, anxious, overstimulated type? If so, you would do well to emphasize the Calming Mini-Moves presented in chapter 4. That will be the perfect place for you to begin your quest for sounder sleep. Read through the introductory texts for each Mini-Move, look at the photos, and choose the one or two of those Calming Mini-Moves that appeals to you most. Then practice as often as you can until you know your chosen Mini-Moves by heart.

Once you can practice fluently, without consulting the book, try to set aside time at least three times a day for ten minutes or more each time. If you can do more, do it! The Basic Program given in the next section provides a suggested schedule for practice of the Calming Mini-Moves. You can use that as your basic guideline, and augment it according to your own intelligence and intuition, as well as your own felt need. The key thing for the nervous type is to integrate the practice of the Calming Mini-Moves into your daily routine so thoroughly that you become saturated with their relaxing effects, and your life becomes distinctly more peaceful. Later, you can gradually introduce the Lulling Mini-Moves just as is recommended in the Basic Program that follows. The more you can practice those Calming Mini-Moves, the more confident you can be that your subsequent practice of the Lulling Mini-Moves is going to bear the sweet, golden fruit of sleep.

Just Plain Sleepless?

Perhaps you've been reading about the tense and nervous types described in the two preceding sections and thinking, "Nope, that's not me." You may be thinking that you suffer from neither physical tension, which is addressed by the Relaxing Mini-Moves in chapter 3, nor nervousness, anxiety, or overstimulation, which are addressed by the Calming Mini-Moves in chapter 4. Your only problem is that you can't sleep. Therefore, you'll skip right to the Lulling Mini-Moves in chapter 5, and your sleep problems will be solved. Makes sense, right?

Whoa, slow down! Stop right there. I know many of my readers will be tempted to think this way. Every troubled sleeper wants to find the shortest, easiest, most convenient path to natural, restful sleep. You want natural, restful sleep and you want it right away! And I want it for you, too. But there's one thing I want to avoid at all cost: the possibility that, in your drive to find the shortest, easiest, most convenient path to sleep, you will take the shortcut and miss out on the essential features of the Sounder Sleep System, features that give this system its full effectiveness and power.

So, for those of you who are neither the tense nor the nervous type, for those who are just plain sleepless: Have I got a program for you! And, if you *are* a tense or a nervous type, you can follow the advice provided for you above, then use this Basic Program as a guide to further practice. So here we go.

The Basic Program

Step 1. First, learn either L.E.S.S. Is More or Making Room, or both, from chapter 4. Whichever you choose, practice at least two or three times—more if you like. They are designed to restore the natural rhythm and balance of your breath. Since all of the Lulling Mini-Moves depend on that easy, natural breathing, these two provide an indispensable preparation for success with the Mini-Moves. That's true for virtually everyone who lives in this hurried, worried, and harried world of ours.

Step 2. Then, learn either Main Squeeze or a Twist of the Wrists, or both, also in chapter 4. Whichever you choose, review that until you can practice fluently, without having to consult the book. Then, for a good week, or even two, practice twice or three times a day, for ten minutes or more each time. Occasionally, you may wish to substitute one of the other Calming Mini-Moves for Main Squeeze or a Twist of the Wrists. Perhaps you are the brooding type who tends to think obsessively—Things Are Looking Up will help you to reduce the volume of your thoughts. Or maybe you tend to be irritable or easily upset—in that case Touching

Your Heart is a good bet. As always, variety is not only the spice of life, but also the greatest ally of the learning process.

What are the best times to practice your Calming Mini-Moves? First thing in the morning is wonderful—many of us get terribly worked up just anticipating what the new day will bring, and a soothing Mini-Move provides an effective antidote that lasts well into the morning. Late morning, just before lunch, is a great time, too. By then we are ready for a brief respite from the stress of the day, and it's easier to focus on the Calming Mini-Moves with a relatively empty stomach. The rumblings of a full stomach can be quite an impediment to concentration. Late afternoon affords a tranquil mood all its own, as the day winds down and we are just beginning to anticipate the approach of night, darkness, and welcome rest. Then again, just before bedtime is a wonderful time for the Calming Mini-Moves. Done at that time, they help our bodies and minds to establish a clear division between active day and passive, restful night, thus assuring that we remain in sync with those ever-present, natural rhythms that are so essential for healthy sleep. The bottom line is, practice the Calming Mini-Moves often, whenever you can. Not only will your life become sweeter and easier, but you will learn many useful relaxation skills that will enhance your later practice of the sleep-inducing Lulling Mini-Moves in chapter 5. Being more relaxed and peaceful during waking hours sets the scene for sounder sleep.

Step 3. After a week or two of regular practice of the Calming Mini-Moves, you'll be ready to begin learning and practicing some of the Lulling Mini-Moves in chapter 5. They are the ones you're going to use to help yourself get to sleep, or back to sleep if you awaken during the night. Again, read the text, browse the pictures, and find the Lulling Mini-Move that strikes your fancy. Your own intelligence and intuition is your surest guide to what is right for you. You might try a Mini-Move and find that it doesn't suit you—try another. In my workshops and in my private practice, I never encourage anyone to persist in doing a Mini-Move that doesn't suit them. Rather, we always look for the one that is just right for the individual. You should, too.

The Waiting Game

I have already mentioned the Waiting Game. That is the one cardinal rule for practicing the Lulling Mini-Moves that I try to impress upon all my students. And you, dear reader, are no exception. The Waiting Game means that you begin your practice of the Lulling Mini-Moves during waking hours only. Wait, wait, wait. Do not attempt to practice in bed until you can do the Mini-Move from memory, with absolute fluency, comfort, and ease.

For every rule, there's a reason, and here's the reason behind this rule: If you have difficulty falling asleep, bedtime is no picnic. It's bound to be a challenging moment, full of doubt, anticipation, apprehension, fear, and other difficult feelings. You probably think to yourself: What's going to happen? Am I going to be able to sleep? Will I awaken too early? If so, at what time? Will I be able to function at my peak tomorrow? Thoughts and feelings such as these tend to be arousing all by themselves. They can wake you right up! Practicing a new and unfamiliar exercise is also arousing, all by itself. Bring the two together, and you've got twice the arousal, so the odds are stacked against falling asleep. Conversely, if you wait until you have really mastered your chosen Mini-Move, until you can practice it with pleasure and ease, and until you have proven its power to yourself many times over during waking hours, then you can gradually introduce that

Mini-Move whenever you need it, be it bedtime, later at night, or early in the morning. Rather than producing arousal, it will deliver you to the shores of sleep. This is the way to achieve sublime success in your quest for sounder sleep.

If you're one of those folks who fall asleep easily at bedtime, but have difficulty staying asleep through the night, the Waiting Game will be even more helpful for you. When you awaken at 3 or 4 or 5 a.m., the most important thing you can do is to remain calm. Do not stir yourself! Do not open your eyes wide, clench your fists, curse your fate, or do anything that is likely to increase your arousal. That will only increase the odds against your getting back to sleep. By the same token, do not attempt to practice a Mini-Move that is unfamiliar or that you can't yet do fluently. It may have the paradoxical effect of waking you up even further. Again, play the Waiting Game.

For you, the Waiting Game actually has two stages that, happily, can make your practice of the Mini-Moves all the more effective. In the first stage, you practice the Mini-Move of your choice for a week or two *during waking hours only*, until you achieve complete fluency. Later, you can practice for a few nights *at bedtime only*. Get into bed, douse the lights, get comfortable, and then, after about ten minutes of quiet rest, begin to do your chosen Mini-Move. That gives you the advantage of practicing your Mini-Move under realistic, nocturnal conditions. But, since you don't expect any trouble falling asleep at bedtime, the pressure is off. The gentle, soothing Mini-Move will effortlessly usher you along the path from waking to sleep. And each time you walk that path, you are training your mind and body to fall asleep in response to those movements. Later, you can practice that same Mini-Move should you awaken during the night. Then you'll have an effective tool that you can use to recover from those unwanted late-night or early-morning awakenings.

Further Advice and Guidance

You will read additional advice and guidance about how to learn and practice each of the three types of Mini-Moves in the next three chapters. What follow are general tips for home practice that I give all my students.

No effort. Make no effort to fall asleep! After all, sleep is the antithesis of effort. Sleep begins with the cessation of all effort. Simply allow these gentle, synchronized movements and breathing to deliver you to the shores of sleep. Once you arrive there, just relax and enjoy the scenery. Allow the innate wisdom of your own mind and body to decide what happens next.

Go with the flow. Remember that there is a broad spectrum of mind-body states between full waking and deep sleep. *In some of the lighter stages it is possible that you may remain aware of your surroundings, leading you to believe you're awake.* Do not be concerned. Those lighter stages of sleep are restful in themselves—far more restful than pacing the floor!—and they are the doorway to deeper, fully restorative sleep. In your gradual descent into sleep, you may drift, you may dream, you may have unusual thoughts or perceptions—that's all part of the slow, step-by-step process of falling asleep. Do allow that natural process to take its course. *Go with the flow.*

Don't shoot. If at bedtime you're not falling into a deep sleep as quickly as you think you should, or if you awaken during the night, you may say to yourself, "Oh, shoot!" or words to that effect. Don't! That vigorous expression of displeasure can wake you up even more. Instead, remain calm, keep on doing your Mini-Moves, with longer and longer rest periods between the movements. *Rest assured,* you'll lull yourself back to sleep step by step.

Don't shoot, part 2. Later in the night, after you've been asleep a while, you may enter a lighter stage of sleep, or even fully awaken. In that case, too, you may say to yourself, "Oh, shoot!" or words to that effect. Don't! That vigorous expression of displeasure wakes you up even more and delays your return to sleep. Instead, do not be concerned—you have prepared yourself for this moment by learning the Mini-Moves. Do them! Little by little, the gentle, synchronized movements and breathing will deliver you to the shores of sleep.

Two steps forward, one step back. The descent into sleep is not a one-way process. It's reversible! You may drift in and out of sleep several times before you really "drop off" into a deeper sleep. Don't resist! Just relax, and let Mother Nature, and the Mini-Moves, take their course. You'll go two steps forward, toward sleep, and one step back, toward waking. Your net gain is one step *forward*. After a couple of rounds of that, you'll find that you've entered a state of deep repose. From there, it's just a hop, skip, and a jump to Slumber Land.

Don't get into a rut. Practice a variety of Mini-Moves. The more variety you can achieve, the more likely you are to find the Mini-Move that's just right for you tonight, and every night. When you begin, practice one or two Mini-Moves of each type that you've mastered. As your practice develops, try to learn the other Mini-Moves and gradually incorporate them all into your regime. Let your own intelligence and intuition be your guide.

Go easy. If you encounter any obstructions in your learning or practice of the Mini-Moves, back off. You can always stop for a few days and begin again fresh. The Calming Mini-Moves L.E.S.S. Is More and Making Room are always a good place to start anew.

General Tips for Sounder Sleep

In addition to your daily practice of the Relaxing, Calming, and Lulling Mini-Moves it's essential that you maintain a peaceful, sleep-supportive lifestyle. Here are some helpful tips to guide you.

Go to sleep at the same time every night. Consistent bedtimes promote a healthy, regular sleep-wake rhythm. This is one of the most important steps you can take to promote sounder sleep.

Take sun. Bright sunlight in the morning also helps to maintain a normal sleep-wake rhythm. It also suppresses daytime melatonin secretion, thereby supporting your full alertness and vigor. If you live in a part of the world where bright sunshine is not regularly available, you might consider getting a light box. This electronic light source provides a "sun supplement" for a half hour or more each day. It can make a big difference during those long, dark winters. My favorite is the LiteBook (available from litebook .com). No larger or heavier than a paperback book, I carry it with me whenever I leave sun-drenched New Mexico for darker climes.

Douse the light. Research shows that our sleeping bodies are extremely sensitive to light, even in small amounts. Light pollution and over-lighting are endemic to modern urban and suburban environments, and even the feeble, first rays of dawn can disrupt the fragile architecture of your early morning sleep. For sounder sleep, be sure that your bedroom is truly dark. Blackout curtains—or at the very least a sleep mask that blocks light from entering your eyes—are a must. Also eliminate from your bedroom all internal sources of light, such as illuminated clocks, computers, or appliances with glowing or blinking LEDs. (Nightlights, if required for safety, should be well out of sightlines from your bed.)

Exercise regularly. Daily exercise appropriate to your physical condition is invigorating, lifts your spirits, and helps promote natural, restful sleep. Working out at the same time every day helps to establish a healthy, sleep-wake rhythm.

Exercise early. Late-night workouts stimulate arousal mechanisms which can delay the onset of sleep. Vigorous exercise causes your body to secrete stress hormones that can keep you awake. Solution: Exercise early in the day. Keep evening workouts light. Avoid exercise within three hours of bedtime.

Don't trade sleep for exercise. Dragging yourself out of bed an hour early for that bleary-eyed workout might seem like a shortcut to better health and fitness, but it can shortchange your sleep needs. And that isn't good for your health. Solution? Enjoy that extra hour of sleep, and reschedule your workout at lunch or just after work.

Subjective insomnia. People often think they're awake when they're actually asleep. It's called *subjective insomnia.* While you may think you're lying awake for hours, you may actually be asleep a good part of that time. Take heart! You may be getting more sleep than you think.

Caffeine blues? The effects of caffeine can last for up to eighteen hours. Caffeine suppresses the natural hormone melatonin, which is essential for evoking sleep onset, and stimulates secretion of stress hormones like cortisol and ACTH, which can keep you awake. Reduce your consumption of caffeine products (including coffee, tea, *chocolate,* and colas) to a minimum. If you must use caffeine, do it as early in the day as possible.

Drowsy driving is no joke. According to sleep research pioneer Dr. William Dement, drowsiness is not an early warning system—it's a red alert! Drowsiness is the last thing that happens before you fall asleep. If you feel drowsy while driving, pull over immediately and rest. Once you feel fully awake, continue your trip safely.

Overwork, under-sleep. Americans work longer hours than any other nation, and we're experiencing an epidemic of sleep deprivation. And the more we work, the less we sleep, according to recent research. If you work more than forty hours a week and aren't getting the sleep you need, consider cutting down on your working hours. You'll sleep better, look better, feel better, and be more creative and productive. Your body will thank you!

Taking the red eye? A study of Long Island Railroad commuters conducted by Joyce Walsleben of New York University concluded that the longer your commute to work, the less sleep you are likely to get. There are only so many hours in the day, and sleep is the first casualty of an overloaded schedule. Possible solutions include changing jobs, moving closer to work, or working from home. Your good health is more important than any job!

Early to bed, early to rise. Grandma was right! The later you go to bed, the later you'll need to sleep. But those extra hours you get by "sleeping in" may not be as restful as you would like. That's because the circadian clock, which synchronizes your body with the rhythms of night and day, boosts your blood pressure and the hormone cortisol starting at around 7 in the morning. That tends to make your sleep shallower and more fragmented. The answer? Get to bed by eleven, and wake up around 7. Just like Grandma said!

Dim the screen. Computers, e-mail, the Internet, and video games are stimulating, whether you feel it or not. If you use a computer close to bedtime, you may experience a considerable delay in sleep onset. Solution: Turn off the computer two hours before your ideal bedtime. Sweet dreams!

Watch what you eat. What and how you eat can significantly influence your sleep. Small and balanced meals, eaten slowly in a quiet environment, are conducive to sound sleep. Rich, greasy, overly spiced foods; overeating; late meals; or a chaotic dining environment can set you up for a night of tossing and turning.

Chapter 3

⋆ ⋆⋆⋆ ⋆

Relax Your Body

The message of this chapter is: Movement matters! The quality of your movement is a key to the quality of your life. By that I mean, the way you *move*—the way you sit, stand, walk, climb stairs, reach for the phone, tap the keyboard, swing a golf club or tennis racket, or carry a baby—has a tremendous impact on how you *feel* and how you *do* in all your daily activities, *including sleep*.

Light, easy, well-coordinated movements feel good and are good for you. They produce feelings of physical and mental ease, self-assurance, and pleasure. They provide a basis for happy and creative living. And most important for our purposes, they *relax* your body and reduce *stress*, which as you know is the number one enemy of sleep. Anything that makes your life less stressful is going to support your quest for more peaceful sleep.

Now consider the other side of the coin. Awkward, ill-coordinated, overly forceful movements feel heavy and uncomfortable. The misdirected effort of the movement rebounds on the body, damaging muscles, bones, and other sensitive tissues. The end result can be stiffness, aches and pains, premature fatigue, low mood, and reduced ability and achievement. Living this way is stressful. The more stress there is in our lives, the harder it is to get a good night's sleep.

So movement does matter. And happily, we've got a choice. Whether we are young or old, weak or strong, healthy or ill, we can always improve the quality of our movements. Using our own senses as a guide, we can become aware of old, habitual ways of moving that don't work and replace them with new ones that do. And it doesn't have to be a big deal. Often, a relatively small change in the way we move can bring a meaningful change in our quality of life. Later, we may choose to make further, deeper changes. In this way can we improve our lives step by step.

A Path to Meaningful Change

How can we make these meaningful changes in ourselves? The best way that I have found is something called the Feldenkrais Method. Created by the Israeli physicist, engineer, and judo master Dr. Moshe Feldenkrais (1900–1984), this fascinating and highly effective method of *movement education* is taught by over six thousand practitioners worldwide and is enjoyed by millions of people from every walk of life. Students of the method enjoy better posture, breathing, and coordination as well as greater mental and physical flexibility. They typically report enhanced performance, creativity, and pleasure in activities as diverse as walking, skiing, dancing, running, golfing, gardening, mathematics, the arts, and business.

What kind of people study the Feldenkrais Method? People like *you*. For example, Feldenkrais helps people with backaches, injuries, or muscle and joint pain to discover new options for easier, more pleasurable movement. This was confirmed by studies conducted by the Santa Barbara (California) Regional Health Authority and at a Saab factory in Sweden. In the Santa Barbara study, Feldenkrais teacher and author Steven Shafarman taught an intensive two-week program for a small group of chronic pain patients with various musculoskeletal and stress-related conditions, including chronic back pain, migraine, and physical trauma. Data from a questionnaire compiled by the American Academy of Pain Management showed that the Feldenkrais program was more effective than standard treatment protocols at about one-tenth the cost. Participants' medical costs declined by roughly 40 percent in the year following this program.

The Saab study, reported in the *Journal of Occupational Rehabilitation,* was designed to investigate whether physiotherapy or Feldenkrais training resulted in a reduction of complaints from the neck and shoulders among ninety-seven female workers. Researchers measured range of motion in neck and shoulders, oxygen consumption, endurance, and physiological capacity according to a dynamic endurance test. Each worker was assigned to one of three groups: One received standard physical therapy (PT) and ergonomic intervention, another received Feldenkrais movement education, and a control group received no intervention. The physical therapy and Feldenkrais program lasted sixteen weeks each during paid work time. Results? The Feldenkrais group "showed significant decreases in complaints from neck and shoulders and in disability during leisure time." The PT group showed no change, while a worsening of complaints was recorded in the control group.

But Feldenkrais isn't just for people in pain. Countless athletes, musicians, and dancers use the method to "fine-tune" their bodies for competition or performance. My friend and colleague Peff Modelski, for example, is a thirty-year veteran of professional ballet who was in the original company of *Fiddler on the Roof* with Jerome Robbins, has been a rehearsal mistress for both the American Ballet Theater and the Joffrey Ballet, and teaches at Steps on

Broadway, NYC's premier professional ballet studio. (On top of all these accomplishments she is also a first-rate teacher of the Sounder Sleep System and the Feldenkrais Method!) Peff has eagerly integrated Feldenkrais into her unique methods of teaching and training dancers. "The method," says Peff, offers dancers "a highly refined awareness of detail and timing, and reestablishes their relation to the ground, to gravity, and to themselves." Prisca Winslow Bradley, another seasoned dance professional, teaches an annual summer workshop in Taos, New Mexico, employing the Feldenkrais Method to train teachers of ballet and modern dance in injury-prevention strategies for their students.

Musicians? Pianist Andrew Rangell, considered one of America's best interpreters of Beethoven and Bach, credits Feldenkrais with his complete recovery from a career-stopping repetitive strain injury. Spain's classical guitar virtuoso Narciso Yepes experienced a similar result after several lessons with Dr. Feldenkrais. Baltimore's Aliza Lidovsky Stewart, no mean pianist herself and a passionate embodiment of Feldenkrais principles, ministers to the artistic aspirations and injuries of musicians in the Baltimore Symphony Orchestra and other musical organizations. Berkeley, California's Mary Spire, another classical pianist turned Feldenkrais teacher, works her movement magic for string, woodwind, and piano players at the Tanglewood Festival every summer. Bob Chapra is a longtime faculty member of Philadelphia's Curtis School of Music, where he teaches the Feldenkrais way to self-awareness to aspiring vocalists and instrumentalists. And let's not forget Willie Nelson, whose daughter Lana describes the result of two Feldenkrais lessons in her online journals: "With one session both hands were 50% better, and today, after [the Feldenkrais teacher] showed up again in Vegas at the House of Blues, Dad's hands were 100% better. No soreness, no stiffness, no swelling, nothing. . . . Trigger [Willie's equine nickname for his famously battered guitar] is saddled up and ready to go. What a wonderful Christmas present!"

Athletes? Sports-related injuries left Carrie Edwards, a world-class rower who had won six national gold medals in rowing between 1990 and 1993, unable to train at a professional level. Feldenkrais teacher Ofer Eretz helped Carrie get back at the oars in time for the 1996 Olympic trials. "I am now training for the next Olympic events with no major obstacles relating to injuries," Edwards comments in an online article by Ruth Jaeger. "As extra benefits I have noticed that my running has become easier, my performance on exercise machines has improved, and my recovery time is easier and shorter. All this without additional training!"

"I can't say enough good things about the Feldenkrais Method!" exults Chris Boyd, former U.S. national track champion. "I believe it has made the difference between continuing my competitive running career and retiring prematurely." Tony Trear, teaching tennis pro and former pro player, says, "The Feldenkrais Method has given me the ability to do things in tennis I could never do before and has relieved my body of the pain accumulated from over twenty years of competitive playing." Basketball great Julius "Dr. J." Erving was an enthusiastic student of Dr. Feldenkrais himself. And PGA Tour veteran Duffy Waldorf says, "The Feldenkrais Method has allowed me to play pain-free golf, without worrying about injury." Feldenkrais teacher Bonnie Kissam has devised an ingenious, recorded program for golfers titled *The Effortless Swing*.

Feldenkrais also helps people young and old with stroke, multiple sclerosis, Parkinson's, and neurological disorders to find more effective ways to get along in daily life. Anat Baniel, an Israeli who worked side by side with Dr. Feldenkrais for the last years of his life, is legendary for her successes with babies and children suffering from severe birth injuries, disease, and developmental disabilities. In an interview in the Feldenkrais Guild publication *Senseability*, Baniel describes her work with a five-year-old girl with muscular atrophy disease. "She was wearing a brace, could not sit herself up from a lying position, and walking was difficult," Baniel recounts. "By the fifth visit she had learned to sit up by herself . . . She's doing things now that were out of her reach and even beyond her imagination." At the University of Heidelberg, Chava Shelhav, who began her apprenticeship with Moshe in Israel in the early fifties, introduced a Feldenkrais-based program for first-grade students with learning disabilities entitled "Movement As a Model for Learning." The class received daily Awareness Through Movement lessons for six weeks. By the end of the year, the class showed significant improvement in posture, balance, and coordination. But the benefits of Feldenkrais are more than merely physical. Baniel says that as children acquire an expanded sense of possibilities in movement, their self-esteem and motivation improve as well. Shelhav echoes this sentiment, noting that the Heidelberg class went on to become one of the most academically advanced classes in the school, and a favorite of the teachers. There was a vibrant social atmosphere in the class, allowing for effortless integration of troubled children entering from other schools. A class used for comparison showed no changes in social structure or apparent learning ability.

This is just a quick survey of what Dr. Feldenkrais and his students have achieved. Success stories like these are known to every Feldenkrais teacher and student. The truth is, Feldenkrais can help anyone, no matter what their age or physical condition, to feel better, perform better at work and play, relax, and enjoy life more. (To locate a Feldenkrais teacher near you, please contact the Feldenkrais Guild of North America, listed in appendix A, and explore some of the other Feldenkrais-related resources listed there.)

Using Your Own Senses for Learning and Growth

What makes the Feldenkrais Method so special? What distinguishes it from other methods of movement education? What accounts for its unparalleled ability to facilitate enhanced learning, performance, and healing in so many different arenas? For me, it's this: Rather than asking you to conform to some predetermined idea of what is best in posture, movement, or coordination, Feldenkrais teaches you how to *use your own senses* to discover the movements that work best for you, in the moment. Instead of showing you one correct way to perform a given action, the Feldenkrais teacher guides you to discover multiple *options for action*. As a result, you become supremely adaptable, so you can respond effectively to rapidly changing, unfamiliar, or unexpected situations. In other words, the Feldenkrais Method sets you free. Free to respond spontaneously, in the moment, to whatever life tosses at you. That's a great way to live.

You see, at birth we humans aren't endowed with the ability for purposeful movement. A calf is born, and it walks immediately. A whale is born, and it swims. But a human being must undergo a long apprenticeship in movement before he or she will sit, stand, or walk. Our brains develop as our bodies grow, and that development and growth drives us to learn and discover more and more each day. And each wondrous discovery—rolling over, lifting one's head, sitting up, crawling, speaking one's first word—brings new information back to the brain, thereby advancing its development even further.

Once we have acquired the movement basics, we go on to refine those skills and abilities in unique and very personalized ways that, to a great degree, define who we are as people. The vast vocabulary of actions and expressions that any adult human being is able to perform is primarily a result of what that person has *learned* in the course of his or her life. Our virtually endless capactiy for *learning as we grow* is one of the greatest faculties of the human species. It has enabled us not only to adapt and survive, but to thrive on this planet. It has enabled all of our positive achievements in art, industry, and culture.

Developing an awareness of how differences in movement make a difference in our lives, and adjusting our behavior accordingly, is one of the hallmarks of human learning. From amongst the infinitude of possible actions, we seek those that best suit our intentions, bringing us the results we want with the least possible effort. Whenever we achieve that, even if only for a moment, we feel pleasure and satisfaction. And that pleasure and satisfaction guide us to further successful action. That is how we learn to move; and that is how we learn to live.

Variety and Spontaneity

Variety is an essential component of healthy movement. When we know only one way to perform an action, we don't have any other choice. We will do what we know whether it suits our needs or not. That is called *compulsive* behavior. But when we have at our disposal a variety of effective ways to perform a given action, we can choose the one that suits us best, in the moment. That way, we can constantly adapt ourselves to our ever-changing environment. This is called *spontaneity*.

Does it really matter whether our actions are compulsive or spontaneous? It matters a lot. On one level, it is a purely practical matter, because compulsive actions often do not produce the results we intend, especially in the rapidly changing circumstances typical of modern life. But this practical issue has broad psychological ramifications because, to the extent our actions are compulsive, we won't know how to get what we want in life. We have all known people who consistently act against their own best interests, and then bemoan the fact that the world isn't fair. They are at war with themselves, and at war with society. This is a classic outcome of compulsive behavior.

Compulsive action also directly undermines our physical well-being. Whenever we perform an action that isn't well suited to the situation at hand, the misdirected effort of that action rebounds onto our own bodies, producing strain. Whenever there is strain, we experience irritation, pain, and disability. By contrast, truly spontaneous action is always easy, graceful, and pleasurable. The effort made is spent entirely on the movement. There is no wasted energy, no strain. When we move that way, life is easy and enjoyable. Instead of wasting our energy on poorly coordinated actions, we have energy to spare for creative pursuits, for love, for meaningful work and play.

It is worth noting that spontaneous movements are not only pleasurable to do, but they are also a joy to watch. If you have ever observed a top athlete, a graceful dancer or skater, a highly skilled surgeon, or even a very good waiter or bartender, then you have already known this to be true. Watching a performance like that causes us to feel the stirrings of spontaneity and pleasure in ourselves, for we are all fully capable of achieving it, too. Isn't life grand?

Incidentally, Dr. Feldenkrais always insisted that this same principle of spontaneity, which is here presented as an aspect of physical movement and coordination, could and should be applied to all our types of thought, action, and expression. "The movements are nothing," he would exclaim, "I'm not after flexible bodies, but flexible brains!" This means that the structured method of self-observation, self-discovery, and self-transformation that is modeled in each Feldenkrais movement lesson is fully applicable not only to the realm of the moving body, but to the intellectual, emotional, and expressive aspects of our being. The full ramifications of that assertion are still being explored and elaborated by Dr. Feldenkrais's many followers.

Guidelines for Practice of Relaxing Mini-Moves

The Relaxing Mini-Moves in this chapter are offered as a specialized application of the Feldenkrais Method rather than a general introduction to the method. They serve three related functions. First, they will help you relax your body and relieve the accumulated physical stress of the day so you can sleep more easily at night. Second, they will introduce you to principles of movement awareness that are essential for effective practice of the Calming and Lulling Mini-Moves presented in chapters 4 and 5. Third, they will introduce and clarify certain movements that might otherwise be unfamiliar to you when you approach those later chapters. The Calming Mini-Moves comprise an essential element of the insomnia solution presented here.

There are six Relaxing Mini-Moves in this chapter. The first three are done lying down. Lying down allows you to explore movements in the absence of your habitual responses to gravity. As a result, the parts of ourselves that most often become stuck or fixated from excess tension in standing or sitting—the muscles of the back, neck, or shoulders are typical examples—can then be mobilized in new and unexpected ways. Later, when we return to standing or sitting, we will find that the habitual tension is alleviated, and we will move with greater ease and efficiency.

When you first practice these Mini-Moves, it is best to lie on an exercise mat or rug on the floor or some other firm surface. A firm yet comfortable surface gives you clearer feedback about your movements than a soft mattress does. Later, if you prefer to do the Mini-Moves while lying in bed, that is perfectly acceptable. If you are bedridden or cannot get down to the floor for any reason, don't let that stop you! In that case, you may practice in bed. (Of course, check with your health care provider to make sure you are well enough to do light exercise. If you are cleared for light exercise, then you can certainly do Mini-Moves.)

The remaining three Relaxing Mini-Moves are done in sitting position. They address issues of general interest but are especially important for anyone who spends long hours sitting at a desk or computer, which includes over 75 percent of all working Americans. Sitting all day is extremely stressful. Lactic acid builds up in your tissues, gravity causes blood pooling in the lower extremities, and muscles get tense and stiff as a result of prolonged immobilization. Computers add another layer of stress to the equation, owing to the exceptional demands they place on the hands and eyes, neck and shoulders. Therefore, anything you can do to make prolonged sitting easier and more comfortable is bound to relieve some of the stress of life. Then you can relax and enjoy life even more.

For the seated Mini-Moves you'll need a stable, standard-height chair or stool with a firm, flat seat. Avoid overly padded chairs; they make it too hard to sense the contact between the chair seat and your bottom. Casters and swiveling seats, as are common on most desk chairs, are not ideal either. These Mini-Moves are meant to help you develop a keener sense of the movements of your body. If the chair rolls or the seat spins it will be that much harder to notice the subtleties of your own movement. So look for a good, old-fashioned chair, the kind with four legs, a firm seat, and a back. Actually, a back is not absolutely required, unless you feel you'll need to lean on it when you rest between movements. The rest of the time, you'll be encouraged to sit on the front half of the seat, without leaning back. That way you will be able to discover your body's full range of seated movement.

When should you practice these Relaxing Mini-Moves? Whenever you like. When you're getting started, the best time will be any time you have a quiet, undisturbed thirty to forty-five minutes or more ahead of you. Later, when you've become more familiar with a Mini-Move, you can review it to good effect in just a few minutes, any time you like. That's particularly true of the seated practices, which can be done right at your desk or workstation whenever you feel the need to inject a little extra mobility, vitality, and self-awareness into your workday. The most important thing is to choose the time that is most practical, convenient, and enjoyable for you.

How often should you practice? As often as you can. For the purposes of our insomnia solution, I would like to see you practice *at least* one of these Relaxing Mini-Moves each week, and briefly review the movements occasionally at other times. (You will be busy with other techniques from chapters 4 and 5 during that time, as well, so you'll have plenty to keep you occupied.)

Anything else you need to know about the Relaxing Mini-Moves is contained in the Mini-Moves themselves. Take your time, keep an open mind, and you will have an enjoyable and relaxing experience. Remember, being more relaxed during waking hours sets the scene for sounder sleep.

Relaxing Mini-Move #1: The Pelvic Rock

> [I]nsomnia is always accompanied by a sense of residual tension and can always be overcome when one successfully ceases to contract the parts in this slight measure.
>
> —EDMUND JACOBSEN,
> *Progressive Relaxation*, 1929

It is said that after the common cold, back pain is responsible for more doctors' visits than any other ailment. (Insomnia is almost certainly third on the list.) Yet many of us have very little sense of what our back is for, how it works, or how to use it in a safe and efficient way. To add injury to insult, the conditions of modern life are far from conducive to a healthy back. The original blueprint for humanity describes active, infinitely adaptable beings capable of an endless variety of actions from the most vigorous—running, jumping, climbing—to the most refined—making sophisticated tools, expressing ideas and emotions, creatively interacting with nature.

But modern life has trapped this multitalented creature in a box of his own making. The chair, the office cubicle, the keyboard, the telephone, the couch, and the car seat, and all the other implements of the sedentary life- and work style offer a sadly diminished scope of action that leaves our bodies crying out for more—more movement, more breath, more variety, more *life*. The backache, the bane of modern man and woman, is one of those cries.

The solution to this nearly universal problem is not a simple one, although the process of self-healing can bring tremendous satisfaction, relief, and pleasure. It typically requires a thorough reeducation of the human frame, which includes the ideas and images we have of our bodies and how they are meant to move. It may also require alterations in one's work and living environment as well as a careful reconsideration of one's priorities in life. That is the subject of another book.

However, there is no denying that the crisis of the back and the crisis of sleep are closely allied, and to address the latter, we must do something about the former. A tense, overworked, unbalanced back and spine can be a major contributing factor in insomnia. Excess muscular tension in the back and the pain that often accompanies it send powerful arousal signals to the brain via the sensory nerves. That excessive arousal can delay the onset of sleep considerably. It can also induce unwanted awakenings during the course of the night.

One of the easiest and most effective ways to work with an overburdened back is to start with the hips and pelvis. You see, our upright posture is not a static structure like a mast or a tower. Rather, it is a dynamic system that constantly adjusts itself in response to the forces acting upon it as we live, move, and breathe. Each component of the postural system has its own special role to play in producing this effect. The hips, encircled as they are by the most powerful muscles in the body, are meant to provide a strong, stable, yet freely mobile base of support for the back and spine. If our hips are stiff, rigid, or poorly coordinated with the whole, a key link in the postural chain is broken. As a result, the muscles of the back, neck, and shoulders have to work overtime to hold the body upright, and we experience the all-too-familiar symptoms that send so many millions of us to the doctor. If our hips are free to assume their natural range of movement, however, and if we know how to utilize the resulting freedom and power of the pelvis to facilitate easy, light, dynamic movement of the whole frame, then we can sit, stand, and walk upright with minimal effort and maximal power, just as nature intended us to do.

The first step in freeing the hips is to bring one's awareness there and explore and clarify the basic movements the hips can make. The traditional Feldenkrais approach is a guided movement process called the Pelvic Clock, in which you lie on your back and slowly rock your hips fore and aft, then side to side, and finally in a series of overlapping arcs, as if your hips were traversing the circumference of an imaginary clock face on the floor. The classic exposition of the Pelvic Clock is in Dr. Feldenkrais's best-known book, *Awareness Through Movement,* and it is a staple of every introductory course in the Feldenkrais Method. For our purposes, a simpler variant is sufficient. I call it the Pelvic Rock.

Here, you'll learn to rock your hips forward and back in a gentle, rhythmic action that ultimately engages the whole body in a delicious, tension-relieving pulsation. When you're done, you may notice welcome changes in your standing and sitting posture and in your gait. And when bedtime comes you'll find that your back, instead of working overtime, can take the night off!

These same movements of the hips will appear in a slightly different context in Rocking the Cradle, a Lulling Mini-Move you'll be learning in chapter 5. Familiarize yourself with the movements now, and when you encounter them later on, your learning will be easy and fun.

Step 1. *Observe yourself at rest.* Lie on your back on a soft mat or carpet on the floor. What are you aware of when you lie quietly like that?

- Notice all the parts of yourself that touch the floor. What is the quality of the contact between your body and the floor? Do you fully relax, allowing the floor to support you? Or are there parts of yourself that feel tense or contracted? The parts of yourself that tend to overwork when you're standing or sitting may take a little longer to come to repose.
- Pay particular attention to the way your bottom, your lower back, your midback, and your shoulders make contact with the floor.
- Notice the point of contact between your head and the floor. Is it high up near the crown of your head, low down near the base of your skull, or somewhere in the middle? Is it on the midline of your skull, or off to one side?
- Notice all the parts of yourself that move as you breathe.

Step 2. *Home position.* Bend your knees and put your feet standing, with the soles of your feet flat on the floor. What is the most comfortable placement for your feet? How far apart would you like them to be? Would you like to have them a little closer to you, or a little farther away? Try to place them in the manner that requires the least effort to maintain.

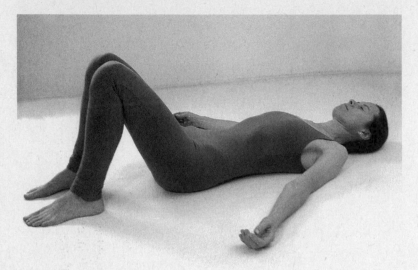

HOME POSITION. Lie on your back. Bend your knees and put your feet standing, with the soles of your feet flat on the floor.

Step 3. *Tilt your hips back.* Very slowly tilt your hips a little bit so that the lowermost tip of your tailbone lifts upward, toward the sky. At the same time, your waist and lower back move downward, toward the earth. Then relax and allow your hips to return to their neutral, resting position. Pause a moment, and then begin again. Repeat the movement slowly, several times. Do small, easy movements.

- Is the movement easy and smooth, or does it feel effortful and uneven? Try to make your movement as smooth and easy as you can.

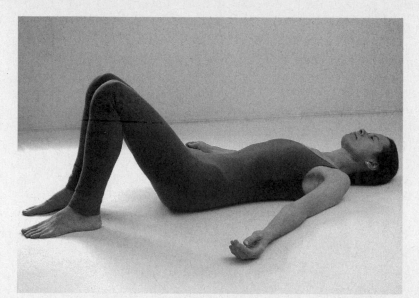

TILT YOUR HIPS BACK. Very gently and slowly, tilt your hips a little bit so that the lowermost tip of your tailbone lifts upward, toward the sky, and your waist and lower back move downward, toward the earth.

- If you experience any strain or feelings of increased effort, stop a moment and rest. Then continue, doing slower, smaller movements.
- If you find that a certain range of the movement is difficult, go back and forth slowly in that range until you can do it easily and pleasantly.
- How do you breathe when you move like that? Do you tend to stop your breath when you do an unfamiliar movement? Can you allow your breathing to be easy and regular?

Step 4. *Stop, rest, and feel.* Straighten your legs and rest. See if you can detect any changes in the way your body makes contact with the floor. Wait until you feel yourself come to a state of repose, then proceed to the next step.

Step 5. *Tilt your hips forward.* This time, slowly and gently tilt your hips the other way. The lowermost tip of your tailbone moves down, toward the earth, and your waist and lower back lift up, away from the floor. Do small, slow, easy movements. Do not strain.

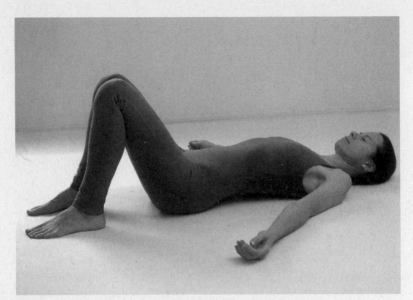

TILT YOUR HIPS FORWARD. This time, slowly and gently tilt your hips the other way. The lowermost tip of your tailbone moves down, toward the earth, and your waist and lower back lift up, away from the floor.

- How does it feel to move your hips that way? Can you make the movement light and easy? Can you allow yourself to breathe freely as you move?
- When you do big, quick, forceful movements, it's hard to tell the difference between a smooth, well-coordinated movement and an awkward one. The sensation of *effort* masks the sensation of the *movement,* just as background noise in a

crowded restaurant makes it hard to hear what's being said at your table.

• With light, easy movement, it's easy to feel even the subtlest differences. You can discover the easiest, most pleasurable way to move. That will enable you to do small movements with exquisite delicacy, big movements with power and precision, and anything in between. You'll be able to adapt your movements quickly to any situation.

Step 6. *Stop, rest, and feel.* You may notice that your back makes a little fuller contact with the floor than before. You may feel as if you were sinking into the floor.

Step 7. *Tilt your hips forward and back.* This time, slowly tilt your hips forward, then tilt them back. Repeat that back and forth movement several times.

As you move like that, notice how your belly moves as you rock your hips forward and back. When you rock your hips forward, does your belly rise up toward the sky or sink down toward the earth? When your hips rock back, does your belly move up, or down?

Notice that your head also moves as you rock your hips. Each time your hips rock forward and the tip of your tailbone moves down, toward the floor, your chin moves in a certain direction. Then, each time your hips rock back and your tailbone rises up toward the sky, your chin moves in response.

Make no effort to move your head, simply observe. The movement of your hips is transmitted through your spine, all the way to your head. Your hips rock, and your head rocks with it. Experiment a little, and see if you can feel the connection between your hips and head.

• Use only that amount of force necessary to move your hips, no more. The movements should be very light and easy.

- Let pleasure be your guide. Light, easy, well-coordinated movements produce pleasurable sensations as your body moves. You feel a sense of comfort and well-being. Awkward, overly forceful movements produce feelings of strain and discomfort.

Step 8. *Stop, rest, and feel.* Straighten your legs and rest a while. Is there any difference in the way your body makes contact with the floor now?

Step 9. *Observe your feet as you rock.* Continue slowly, gently rocking your hips as before.

This time, notice what happens to your feet as you move like that. When your hips rock forward, do your feet get heavier, do they press the floor a little harder? Or do they get a little lighter on the floor? When your hips rock back, do your feet get heavier, or lighter? Repeat the movement several times and see what you discover.

Step 10. *Stop, rest, and feel.*

Step 11. *Rhythmic pulsation.* Now, continue rocking your hips forward and back. But this time, reduce the amplitude of the movement by half. That means, do a movement that is 50 percent smaller than before. Do several smaller, easy movements like that.

Continue, reducing the amplitude of your movement by half again. Do tiny, light, easy movements—the smallest, easiest, most delicate movements you can do with your hips.

Now do the movements quickly—like a series of quarter notes in a waltz. One, two, three; one, two, three; one, two, three; and so on.

Activate your hips only; make no other effort. The gentle, rocking motion of your hips generates a pulsation that spreads through your entire frame. Your feet, legs, back, belly, chest, shoulders, neck, and head all become entrained in the gentle motion. Even your hands and arms get into the act.

Try different speeds: a little faster, a little slower. You can experiment with the amplitude of the movement, too. Find the combination of speed and amplitude that yields the most pleasurable, satisfying pulsation for you. Let your senses be your guide.

What happens to your breath when you pulsate like that?

Step 12. *Stop, rest, and feel.* That gave you a little bit of a workout, didn't it? Now, just observe as your body returns to a state of repose. Rest as long as you like.

Notice again the contact between your body and the floor. You may notice a variety of changes, some small, others more pronounced. Certain parts of yourself that didn't touch the floor when you began may now touch the floor, allowing themselves to be supported by it. Other parts that did touch the floor may make firmer contact with it than before. If so, these are indications of reduced muscular tension and more thorough repose. This is good!

Step 13. *Final observations.* Try the original movements again. A few times, slowly rock your hips forward. See how that feels now. Then, a few times, slowly rock your hips back. How does that feel? You may find that the movements are a little clearer, a little easier, and a little more comfortable than when you began. Those small differences in the quality of your movement can make a big difference in the quality of your life. See what you discover!

Very slowly, without making any sudden movements, roll to one side and stand up. You needn't stretch your arms or legs, or do anything special. Just stand for a moment and feel. Can you feel your hips, your pelvis, while standing? Try rocking your hips a little in that position. As you begin to move about the room, notice any changes in the way you move or the way you feel. Over the next hours or days, you may find yourself doing familiar things in new ways. These movement lessons encourage a process of self-exploration and self-discovery. There is no limit to your potential for learning and improvement.

Relaxing Mini-Move #2: Unlocking Your Rib "Cage"

The 2001 film *Winged Migration* depicts an Amazon river canoe transporting a load of forlorn-looking, captured wild animals to market. One of them, an exquisitely plumed parrot, gets curious about the primitive bolt that locks the door of his cage. Little by little, by deft movements of his head and beak, he teases the bolt open and takes to the air. At the moment of release we breathe a sigh of relief, as if a tremendous weight had been lifted from our chests.

We speak of our ribs as a cage, and they do look like one in anatomy books and on the lifeless skeletons that hang in our science classrooms. For us the living, however, "rib cage" is a truly unfortunate turn of phrase. A cage is something rigid and confining—something locked—and a healthy set of ribs should be anything but. Our ribs are meant to be highly flexible and freely movable. Flexible, movable ribs allow us to breathe and move freely and fully.

Only when we can breathe and move freely and fully can we be truly alive. We perform all our daily activities with the minimum effort necessary. That not only saves a lot of wear and tear on our bodies, but also leaves us more time and energy for creativity, conviviality, self-nurturing, and love. As a result, life is easier, more pleasurable, more peaceful. And as you know, creating a more peaceful life is one of the secrets of sounder sleep.

The Relaxing Mini-Move that follows will help you to achieve greater freedom of movement of your ribs and chest. Follow the instructions step by step, and you'll experience your living, moving body in a whole new way. Then, like our friend the Amazonian parrot, you can unlock your "cage" and regain the freedom and vitality you were born to enjoy.

Step 1. *Observe yourself in action.* Stand up with your arms hanging comfortably at your sides. Then, gently turn and look to the right and to the left several times. Do not stretch or strain; just do what comes easily, without excess effort.

- How does it feel to turn like that? Does it feel easy and light, or heavy and stiff? What parts of yourself participate in the movement? What parts of yourself remain still? Do certain parts of your body seem to limit the movement, preventing you from turning farther? Don't try to change anything at this point; just observe yourself as you turn.
- How far to the right and to the left can you see when you turn like that? As you turn, please make a mental note of some object that you can see to your far right, and another to your far left. That will give you a measure of the range of your movement that you will use for later comparison.

Step 2. *Observe yourself in repose.* Lie on your back on a soft mat or carpet on the floor or other firm surface. Place a firm pillow or a folded blanket under your head for comfort, if necessary. Bend your knees and place the soles of your feet flat on the floor. Rest quietly in that position, and observe yourself.

- What parts of your body make the most distinct contact with the floor? Is it some part of your foot or leg? Is it your buttocks or lower back? Can you feel that certain parts of your back press the floor more distinctly, while others press less so?

OBSERVE YOURSELF IN REPOSE. Lie on your back on a soft mat or carpet on the floor or other firm surface. What parts of your body make the most distinct contact with the floor?

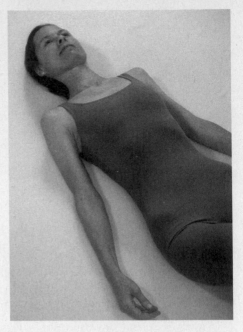

- Pay particular attention to your shoulders as they lie on the floor—your right shoulder, then your left shoulder. How does your right shoulder make contact with the floor? Can you feel it touching the floor, or not? Does it touch the floor at a single point, at several different points, or does it lie flat on the floor like a dinner plate? Does the contact between your right shoulder and the floor feel snug and complete, or does it feel awkward and uncertain?
- How about your left shoulder? Does your left shoulder contact the floor at a point or points, or does it lie snug against the floor? Does your left shoulder make contact with the floor in the same way that your right shoulder does, or are they different?

Step 3. *Float your shoulder.* Slowly, gently lift your right shoulder a little bit off the floor. Move your shoulder very softly, as if it were floating upward on a gentle breeze. Then, gradually allow your shoulder to sink back to the floor. Pause a few moments, allowing the shoulder to come to rest. Then begin again. Repeat several times. Remember to pause after each movement.

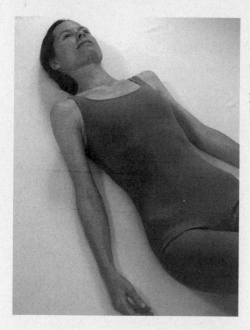

FLOAT YOUR SHOULDER. Slowly, gently lift your right shoulder a little bit off the floor. Then, gradually allow your shoulder to sink back to the floor.

- As you move your shoulder like that, notice any other parts of yourself that move in concert with the shoulder. You will certainly feel your shoulder blade lifting off the floor and then touching down. Can you also feel your right collar bone moving, too? How about your sternum? (Your sternum is the vertical breastbone in the center of your chest, where the ribs are joined together.) Can you identify any physical sensations in your ribs or your back when you move like that? How about your belly or your waist?

Step 4. *Use your hand to monitor the movement.* Bend your left elbow so you can touch your sternum with the fingers of your left hand. Continue floating your right shoulder up and down, while using your left hand to monitor the movements of your sternum. Can you feel your sternum moving a little to one side as you float your shoulder upward, and back to the middle as you float it downward?

- Take your time! Slow, gentle movements allow you to feel yourself as you move. By taking the time to really feel, you will develop a new sense of your self. That will enable you to be more creative and spontaneous in everything you do.

Stop and rest a while. Notice how your right shoulder makes contact with the floor now. Is it different now?

Step 5. *Synchronize your head and shoulder.* Continue as before, slowly floating your right shoulder up and down. Pause to feel the difference after each movement.

- As you do that, do you feel your head tending to roll a little bit to one side? You may experience it as a gentle shifting of the point of contact between your head and the floor, or you may notice a slight change in the direction of your gaze each time you move your shoulder.

Do a few more movements, and now, each time you float your shoulder upward, deliberately roll your head very gently to the left. See if you can find the proportion of shoulder to head movement that feels "just right." Imagine that your shoulder and your head move in perfect unison, as if they were linked by an invisible connecting rod. Repeat that "just right" movement several times, pausing to rest a bit after each repetition.

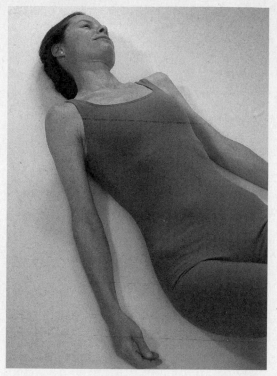

SYNCHRONIZE YOUR HEAD AND SHOULDER. Each time you float your right shoulder upward, deliberately roll your head very gently to the left.

Stop, rest, and feel the effect of what you've done. Notice how your right shoulder makes contact with the floor now.

Step 6. *Float your shoulder again.* Slowly float your right shoulder up and down a few more times. Does the movement feel a little different now? Is it getting lighter, easier, smoother, softer? Can you feel any pleasurable sensations as you move? If so, you're definitely on the right track.

Stop, rest quietly, and feel the effect of what you have done. Feel the difference between your right shoulder and your left, between the right side of your back and the left side of your back, between the whole right side of your body and the left. Does one side feel longer, softer, more at ease? Does one side surrender its weight to the floor more completely?

Step 7. *Imagine your other shoulder.* Lie on your back as before. In your imagination only, do the same slow, gentle floating movements with your left shoulder. Try to imagine all the parts of yourself that would participate in the movement: your shoulder blade, your collar bones, your ribs and sternum, your head and neck.

- Pay particular attention to the movement of your sternum. Try to imagine it accurately. Repeat the imaginary movement many times, until the image of the movement with all of its parts is quite clear in your mind.

Finally, do three or four actual movements of your left shoulder. Slowly float your left shoulder upward, and slowly float it back down to the floor. You may discover that the movement is already, without any actual practice, quite free and easy, quite light and smooth. When your mental image is clear and complete, you can perfect a movement without much practice. The movement naturally conforms to your mental image of it.

Stop, rest, and feel the result of what you've just done.

Step 8. *Rock your shoulders, roll your ribs.* Float your right shoulder up and down one time, then do the same with your left. Repeat that alternating movement many times.

- Allow that alternating movement of the shoulders to generate a slow, rhythmic rolling of the entire rib cage from side to side. Invite every part of yourself to participate in the movement: your head, your ribs, your sternum; your back, waist, and hips. You may even feel your legs and feet begin to respond.

- Relax your forehead, relax your eyebrows, relax your lips, relax your tongue.
- Allow your breath to be very soft and light. You needn't huff and puff. Simply let your breath come and go of its own accord, and you will automatically get just the right amount of oxygen for each moment of your life.

Stop, rest, and feel the result of what you've done.

Step 9. *Unlock your "cage."* Slowly float your right shoulder upward, and as you do so, *very gently* press your left shoulder into the floor. You needn't press hard! Then lower your right shoulder, and stop pressing with the left. Repeat several times. Float the

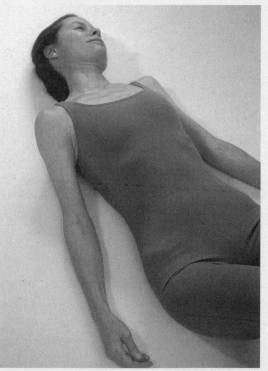

UNLOCK YOUR "CAGE." Slowly float your right shoulder upward, and as you do so, *very gently* press your left shoulder into the floor. You needn't press hard! Then lower your right shoulder, and stop pressing with the left.

right shoulder upward as you press the left shoulder down. After each movement, pause a moment, then begin anew.

- When you do this movement, you will feel your sternum begin to move in a curious trajectory. Does it slide, or twist, or tilt to the left, or is it a combination of all three? Does the upper end of your sternum move in unison with the lower end, or are they slightly out of phase? Did you ever imagine your chest could move like that?

Step 10. *Reverse.* Do the reverse, floating your *left* shoulder and pressing your *right* shoulder to the floor. After each movement, pause a moment, then begin again. Repeat several times, then stop, rest, and feel.

Step 11. *Alternate.* Alternately float your *right* shoulder and press your *left* to the floor; then float your *left* shoulder and press the *right*. Repeat many times, allowing your head, neck, shoulders, and chest to participate in the movement.

- It's a funny sort of a movement, isn't it? Can you feel that the formerly rigid, confining "cage" of your ribs is beginning to become very open, very soft, very pliable? With a splendidly mobile chest like that, who knows what you might accomplish? At the very least, you will gain a different perspective on life. Then, add to that just a dash of that boundless curiosity, ingenuity, and enthusiasm of yours, and, voila!, the world is your oyster!

Stop, rest, and feel. Notice how your left and right shoulder make contact with the floor now. How about the right and left sides of your back? Compare the right side of your body to the left. Does one side feel longer, softer, more at ease? Does one side surrender its weight to the floor more completely? Or do they feel more or less balanced now?

Step 12. *Turn while standing.* Slowly roll to your side and stand up with your arms resting comfortably at your sides. Gently move your right shoulder a little bit forward and back to the starting position. Repeat several times. When you move your shoulder like that, do your head, your ribs, your sternum, and your chest move too? Where do your eyes go?

Step 13. *Left shoulder.* Try the same thing with your left shoulder. Move your left shoulder forward, and allow your head, ribs, sternum, and chest to become engaged. Your left shoulder moves forward, and you turn to the right. What do you see with your eyes?

Step 14. *Right shoulder.* Move your right shoulder forward and, at the same time, move your left shoulder back. Then relax and come back to the starting position. Repeat several times. See if you can utilize your newfound freedom of the chest and sternum when you're standing up, too.

Step 15. *Do the reverse.* Move your left shoulder forward and your right shoulder back. Look for that feeling of freedom in your sternum. Turn and look to your right.

Step 16. *Rhythmic turning.* Now, gently turn and look to the right and to the left several times as you did at the beginning. As before, do not stretch or strain; just do what comes easily, without excess effort.

- How does it feel to turn like that now? Does it feel easy and light, or heavy and stiff? What parts of yourself participate in the movement? What parts of yourself remain still? Can you feel that certain impediments to the movement have been removed and you can turn your body more freely and easily?
- How far to the right and to the left can you see when you turn like that? Can you see only the landmarks you chose at the beginning, or can you see ten or twenty or thirty degrees farther? How far can you see to the right?

Make several more movements, turning your trunk right and left and allowing your arms to swing freely. Allow your chest to be free and flexible. Look for the most pleasurable way to do the movement. Try to keep an even rhythm. Try turning a little faster, then a little slower. What is the most natural rhythm for you? Can you breathe freely and easily as you move like that?

Application. You would be well advised to review these movements of the ribs at regular intervals. Life in our man-made environment is stressful, the ribs are one place where we tend to contract in response. Emotions such as fear, anger, and anxiety can also be contributing factors. You may find that your chest needs a little refresher course from time to time. Now you know what to do to keep it all moving.

Relaxing Mini-Move #3: Lengthening One Side of Your Trunk

What's your trunk? Well, think of a tree. The trunk is the biggest, thickest segment of the tree: everything above the roots and below the branches. You have a trunk, too. It's the main segment of your body: everything above the legs and below the head and neck, excluding your arms. And while a tree trunk is more or less rigid, a human trunk is not. The spine, which is the trunk's central supporting member, is made up of twenty-four jointed segments called vertebrae, and they are made to move. Each joint in the spine makes its own special contribution to our uniquely human posture and movement.

In this Mini-Move you'll expand your awareness of one of the fundamental movements of the trunk. Master it, and you'll find that you move with greater ease and aplomb. If you've ever wanted to dance jazz or Latin, but didn't think you had what it takes, this might help you realize that those limitations are mostly in your mind. Who knows? You might have a whole new career ahead of you! Or not. But sometimes just knowing you could do it if you wanted to is enough to make a difference in the way you feel about yourself. When your movements are easy and light, everyone is a potential partner in the dance of life. Tango, anyone?

This movement is the basis for the Mini-Moves Making Room, in chapter 4, and the Ziggurat, in chapter 5. Get comfortable with the movement now, and learning those later Mini-Moves will be pure pleasure.

Step 1. *Prelude—raise your arms.* Stand up, and slowly raise your right arm to the ceiling without strain, without stretching. Just raise your arm simply, and see how it feels. Does your arm feel light and easy to manage, or heavy and cumbersome? Now do the

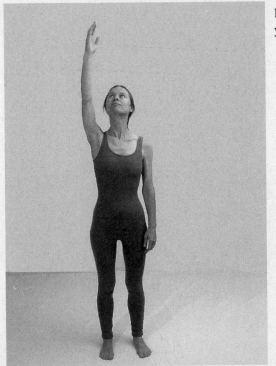

PRELUDE. Raise your arms.

same with your left arm. How does that feel? Make a mental note of it so you'll have something to compare with later on.

Step 2. *Observe yourself in repose.* Lie on your back for a few moments. Notice how the various parts of your body make contact with the floor underneath you. Do you feel that you lie easily and comfortably on the floor, or do certain parts of your body feel awkward or uneasy? Which parts of your body move as you breathe?

Step 3. *Home position.* Please lie on your right side on a soft rug, a blanket, or an exercise mat on the floor. Bend your right arm and put it under your head with your palm up. (If necessary for comfort, you may use a pillow to support your head instead.)

Bend your legs at the hip and knee so that your knees lie on the floor in front of you. The left leg lies on top of the right in a symmetrical fashion. Place your left hand palm down on the floor in front of you.

If you're not able to lie on the floor, lie in bed. A firmer mattress will allow you to sense your movements more accurately than a soft one. However, your comfort and safety should be your first priority, now and always. Do what feels right to you.

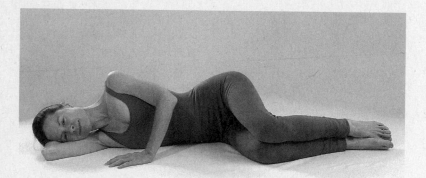

HOME POSITION. Lie on your right side. Bend your right arm and put it under your head with your palm up. (If necessary for comfort, you may use a pillow to support your head instead.) Bend your knees and hips.

- Notice how the ribs on your right side lie against the ground. Are your ribs really at rest there? Do they fully surrender their weight to the ground? Or is there some hesitation, no matter how slight? What about the right side of your waist? Is your waist really at rest, or does it seem to hold back from the floor, even slightly?
- Notice your right hip. Feel the weight of your right hip pressing the ground. What part of your hip presses most distinctly? See if you can find a certain spot where the weight feels most concentrated.

Step 4. *Slide your foot down.* Now, slide your left foot a little bit down, away from your head, as if you were going to straighten your leg. Do not straighten your leg all the way! Just slide your left foot down a little bit, and then come back to the home position. Repeat several times.

- As you move like that, see if you can feel what happens to your left hip. Does your hip move in a certain direction each

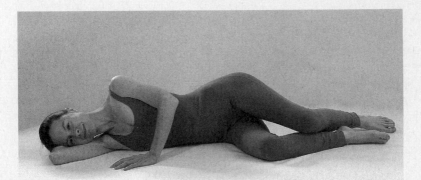

SLIDE YOUR FOOT DOWN. Slide your left foot a little bit down, away from your head, as if you were going to straighten your leg. Do not straighten your leg all the way. As you move like that, see if you can feel how your left hip moves. Then come back to the home position.

time you slide your foot? Place your hand on your left hip and slide your foot a few times more. Can you feel the movement of your hip now?

Step 5. *Stop, lie on your back, and rest.* Notice how your body makes contact with the floor now. How do you breathe? Is your breathing easy and light, or do you huff and puff or hold your breath?

Step 6. *Mobilize your shoulder.* Lie on your right side, as before. Very gently move your left shoulder up, in the direction of your ear. Do several small, easy movements so you can feel and move safely and accurately. As you become accustomed to the movement, you can gradually increase the range little by little.

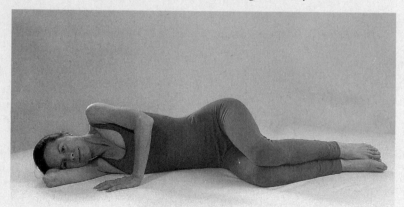

MOBILIZE YOUR SHOULDER. Very gently move your left shoulder up, in the direction of your ear. Then allow the shoulder to come to rest.

- As you move your shoulder like that, what happens to your ribs on your left side? Do they become compressed, or do they spread apart? What happens to the distance between your left shoulder and your left hip? Does it get longer, or shorter when you move your shoulder?

- Continue a few times more. What happens to your ribs on the right side, underneath you? When your shoulder moves up, do the ribs on your right side press into the floor more firmly, or do they get a little lighter? Notice what happens as you return your shoulder to its resting position. Do your ribs press more firmly, or less so, then?

Step 7. *Stop, rest, and feel.* Roll to your back and rest. Does the floor feel the same to you, or different? The changing quality of your contact with the floor gives you valuable feedback about yourself.

Step 8. *Move your hip down.* Lie on your right side, as before. Again, slide the foot down a little bit, as if to straighten your leg.

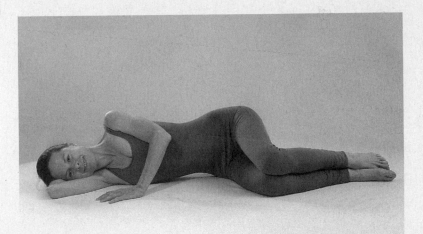

MOVE YOUR HIP DOWN. Move your hip down, away from your shoulder. What happens to your ribs underneath you on the right side? Do they get lighter, as if they would lift off the floor? Or do they press the floor more firmly?

Repeat several times. See if you can feel how your hip moves now. When you slide your foot like that, does your hip move down, away from your shoulder?

Bring your foot back to the home position so your two legs lie parallel. Now, without moving your foot or leg, can you move your hip down, away from your shoulder? Try it several times, without forcing. Just see if the movement is a little clearer to you now. Move your hip alone, down and back, several times. Your leg and your foot stay where they are. It needn't be a large movement. Small is beautiful!

Step 9. *Stop, rest, and feel.* Roll to your back and rest awhile. Allow your breathing to be light and easy. Each time you exhale, that's another opportunity to let yourself sink into the floor a little more.

Step 10. *Elongate your leg.* Roll to your right side as before. This time, straighten your left leg all the way. Raise your leg off the floor a little bit, or, if it's more comfortable for you, let it rest on the floor. In that position, move your left heel downward, away

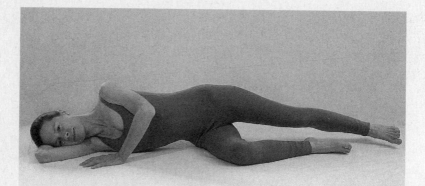

ELONGATE YOUR LEG. Straighten your left leg. Move your left heel downward, away from your head, so that your leg gets longer. Then return to the starting position.

from your head, so that your leg gets *longer*. What can you do with your hip, your lower back, your ribs, your shoulder, to enable that leg to grow longer?

Repeat several times, elongating your leg, and coming back to the starting position. Make the movements easy and light. Don't stretch, don't strain. Try to engage every part of yourself in the movement.

- When you elongate your leg like that, what happens to the ribs that lie underneath you, on your right side? Do they press the floor harder, or do they lighten up? How about your waist? Does it press harder, or does it lighten up? Repeat the movement several times more, and see what you discover.

Then, bend your leg again and return to the home position. Try moving your hip down now. See if the movement is getting a little clearer, a little easier.

Step 11. *Stop, rest, and feel.* Roll to lie on your back for a few moments. Notice how the right and left sides of your body make contact with the floor now. Does one side feel different?

Step 12. *Lengthen one side.* Roll again to your right side. Very gently, move your left hip down, and at the same time move your left shoulder up, toward your ear. Your shoulder and your hip move apart, and the whole left side of your body grows longer. Then rest, and allow your hip and shoulder to return to the home position.

Repeat the movement several times, looking always for the most pleasurable, least effortful way to do it. Don't stretch or strain—make each movement easier and lighter than the last.

Step 13. *Roll to your back and rest for a few minutes.* How long does it take you to regain complete repose after a series of gentle movements like that?

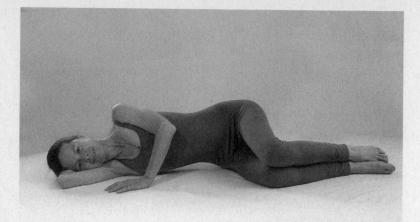

LENGTHEN ONE SIDE. Very gently, move your left hip down, and at the same time move your left shoulder up, toward your ear. Your shoulder and your hip move apart, and the whole left side of your body grows longer.

Step 14. *Feel the difference.* Slowly roll to your side and stand up. Take a moment to see what that feels like now. You may notice that one leg feels a little firmer or more supportive than the other. You may notice that one side of your back feels stronger or more at ease than the other. Perhaps one side of your body feels a little taller than the other.

Slowly raise your left arm toward the ceiling. How does that movement feel now? Raise and lower it a few times, slowly and gently. Does your arm feel lighter and easier to manage than when we began? Try raising your right arm. Which arm feels lighter, longer? Which arm is more at ease?

Step 15. *Explore the other side.* After you've completed Steps 1 through 14, lie down and rest for a while. Then, when you're ready, lie on your left side and repeat all the movements, this time with your right hip and shoulder. Don't hurry. Take your time and see what you discover.

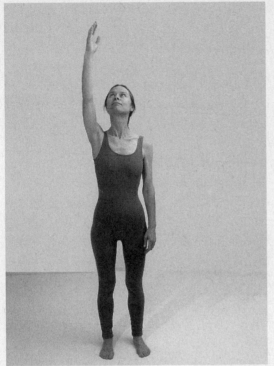

FEEL THE DIFFERENCE. Stand up, and see how that feels. Does one leg feel firmer and more stable? Slowly raise your right arm and lower it. Then your left. Does one arm feel lighter, longer, easier to move now, as compared to when you began?

Relaxing Mini-Move #4: Slouch and Recover

There is nothing wrong with slouching! Like all movements we can do with our bodies, slouching has an honorable place in the repertoire of human action. When you are trying to find an item in your desk drawer, for example, it is quite natural to slouch. When you are *resting* after a period of seated activity, such as writing, drawing, or typing, slouching is the natural way to give the postural muscles of your back and hips a much-needed rest. That's exactly why you do it!

For seated *action*, however, slouching is not the best way to coordinate your body. Generally speaking, a range of upright postures is the safest and most efficient, because these postures provide the greatest mechanical advantage and the greatest freedom of movement for the organs of action—the arms and hands, head and eyes. I say a *range* of upright postures, because healthy sitting is never a matter of assuming a static posture and holding. Rather, we move through a wide range of varied postures according to the level of our activity, our energy, and our attention. This is called *cyclical* sitting.

At moments of intensive activity, the well-coordinated person tends to sit dynamically erect, for that is the *active* posture. As the action slows, the posture tends to relax. When persons pause to think or rest, they may slouch markedly, often reclining against the backrest. At frequent intervals they may perform gentle, enlivening movements in place or stand up and move about in answer to the atavistic need for physical movement. After a pause of the desired duration, the cycle is repeated.

A laboratory simulation of "cyclical sitting" has been studied by a group of researchers at McGill University in Canada. They found that cyclical, dynamic sitting is significantly more comfortable, expends less energy, and produces less stress on the spine than other sitting styles. That's not surprising, because cyclical sitting affords a natural *variety* of movement and posture. As ever, variety is one of the fundamental requirements of our living, moving bodies.

Two recent studies reported in *New Scientist* magazine suggest that chronic, unrelieved slouching may actually damage the supporting muscles of the back. In a study conducted by the European Space Agency in Berlin, researchers studied a group of young male volunteers who spent eight weeks in bed. The study indicates that absence of load on the spinal support muscles may be just as debilitating as physical injuries caused by whiplash or heavy lifting. Another group at the University of Queensland in

Australia studied the same volunteers using magnetic resonance imaging (MRI). It showed that after the eight weeks of enforced bed rest, the multifidus muscles of the back had wasted and become inactive. Subjects monitored for six months after the experiment had still not recovered, even with exercise. They were taught to reactivate the muscles using visual feedback from ultrasound scans.

The following Mini-Move will help you to enliven the muscles of your back using sensory feedback from your own body. In it you will learn to slouch and to recover from a slouch, in a smooth, easy, well-coordinated way. This is one of the fundamental movements that constitute dynamic sitting. As you master this movement, you will find yourself able to sit taller and hold your head up with less effort. And when the time comes to slouch, you can do it with aplomb. Your back muscles will become more pliable, more freely mobile, more alive.

This essential addition to your movement vocabulary can help to relieve much of the physical stress on your neck and shoulders, while freeing up your hands and arms for easier, more inspired writing, keyboarding, mousing, drawing, painting, piano-playing, or any other seated activity.

With a wide variety of well-coordinated movements at your disposal, you will be able to adjust your posture spontaneously according to your ever-changing needs, moment to moment. That's a great way to live. And of course, the reduction in your daily stress quotient sets the scene for sounder sleep. See for yourself!

Step 1. *Observe your sitting posture.* Find a comfortable, stationary chair, preferably one with a flat, horizontal seat pan. Sit on the front half of the seat, any way that you like as long as you are not leaning on the backrest. Place your hands in your lap and your feet on the floor.

OBSERVE YOUR SITTING POSTURE. Sit on the front half of the seat, any way that you like as long as you are not leaning on the backrest.

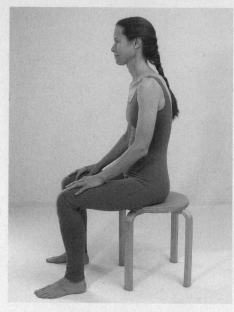

- Take a few moments to notice how you sit. Notice how your buttocks make contact with the chair. Do you place your weight more on the right buttock or the left? Do you sit more on the rearward portion of your buttocks, nearer to the backrest, or more on the forward part, near your thighs? Don't change anything; just observe how you're sitting right now.
- Continue observing your seated posture. Is it easy to hold your head up? Or do your neck and shoulders feel like they are working overtime? Do you feel that you are sitting tall, or does your body feel collapsed, cramped, and contracted?
- Slowly turn your head to the right and left. Is that easy to do, or does the movement feel stiff or limited in some way? Notice your breathing. Do you breathe freely, or do you tend to hold your breath?

Step 2. *Look down.* Sit as before, with your hands in your lap and your feet on the floor. Slowly lower your head and look down to see your belt buckle. (If you're not wearing a belt, just imagine that you are, and look where your belt buckle would be!) Then slowly raise your head and return to the starting position. Repeat several times.

- How do you do this movement? Do you simply incline your head forward by bending your neck, while the rest of your body remains still? Or could you make the movement easier by bringing more of yourself into action?

Step 3. *Engage your ribs and chest.* Continue as before, looking down to see your belt buckle. Perhaps you can sense that each time you lower your head and eyes to look down, your chest tends to tip downward, toward your belly, in concert with the

LOOK DOWN. Slowly lower your head and look down to see your belt buckle.

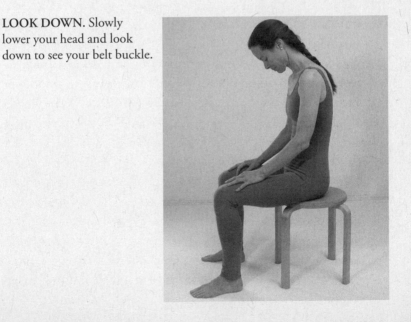

ENGAGE YOUR RIBS AND CHEST. Each time you lower your head and eyes to look down, your chest tends to tip downward, toward your belly. As you raise your head and eyes, your chest rises to help bring the head to the upright position.

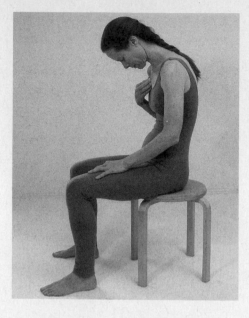

movement of your head and eyes. As you raise your head and eyes, your chest rises to help bring the head to the upright position.

If you are unsure of the movement, place the fingertips of one hand on your sternum, or breastbone, as you do a few of the movements. (The sternum is the vertical bone in the middle of your chest, where the ribs come together.) This will help you to feel what is happening. Once you get a sense of how your sternum and ribs move as you raise and lower your head, you can put your hand back in your lap.

Continue, lowering your head and eyes to look down at your belt buckle, and then sitting up. Each time you go down, move your chest down, too. As you come up, gently raise your chest to help you lift your head. Try to synchronize the movements of your head with the movements of your chest so they begin and end at the same time.

Stop and rest for a few moments. See if you find yourself sitting a little taller than when you started.

Step 4. *Engage your lower back.* Continue as before, lowering your head and chest so you can see your belt buckle, and then sitting up again. Slouch and recover.

You may have already noticed that your lower back (the part of your back just above your waist) tends to move back, toward the backrest of your chair, as you slouch, and forward as you recover. Continue lowering and raising your eyes, head, and chest as before, allowing your lower back to participate as well. Each time you slouch, allow your lower back to move backward. Your back rounds slightly. Each time you recover, allow your lower back to move forward. Your back arches gently. Little by little your entire torso becomes involved in the action.

If you're not sure of the movement, you can place one hand behind you so the back of your hand rests on your back at waist level. That will help you to feel how your lower back moves as you

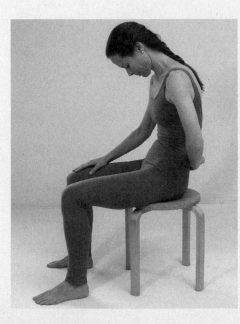

ENGAGE YOUR LOWER BACK. Each time you slouch, allow your lower back to move backward. Your back rounds slightly. Each time you recover, allow your lower back to move forward.

slouch and recover. Then take your hand away and do a few more movements. Is it a little clearer now?

Step 5. *Rock your pelvis.* Notice the changes in the way your buttocks make contact with the chair as you slouch and recover. Lowering your head produces a gentle backward rocking of your pelvis; you sit more on the *rearward* portion of your buttocks. Raising your head produces a gentle forward rocking of your pelvis; you sit more on the *forward* portion of your buttocks.

Gradually you can allow your entire body, including your pelvis, to participate in raising and lowering your head. Pause for a moment. See how you are sitting now.

Step 6. *Put it all together.* The exercise you have just done teaches you to rely on the coordinated action of your chest, trunk, and pelvis to support and mobilize your sitting body. This will make upright sitting easier and more comfortable.

ROCK YOUR PELVIS.
Lowering your head produces a gentle backward rocking of your pelvis; you sit more on the *rearward* portion of your buttocks.

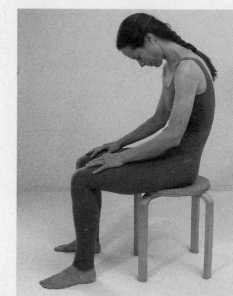

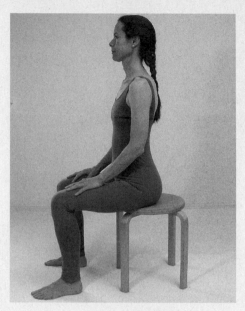

ROCK YOUR PELVIS.
Raising your head produces a gentle forward rocking of your pelvis; you sit more on the *forward* portion of your buttocks.

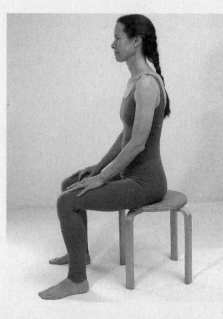

PUT IT ALL TOGETHER.
Pause and observe your seated posture. See if there is any difference, however small, in the way that you sit. You may find that you spontaneously sit a little taller than before.

Slouch and recover a few more times. As you move, try to include each part of yourself—your head and eyes, your chest, your lower back, your pelvis and buttocks—as you have learned. Each part plays its own distinct role in producing a smooth, well-coordinated movement of the whole body.

- Pause and observe your seated posture. See if there is any difference, however small, in the way that you sit. Slowly turn your head to the right and left a few times. Is it a little smoother than when you started this exercise? Perhaps a different part of your bottom is making contact with the chair than when you first observed it. Your breathing may be a little easier. You may find that you spontaneously sit a little taller than before.

Application. As you go about your daily activities, take a few moments each day to repeat some of these movements and to recall what you have learned. There is no need to force yourself to sit in any particular way. Just do what comes naturally. Your posture and movement will begin to change spontaneously, when you are ready. After a few days, you may wish to do this exercise again. It may feel quite different to you the second time around.

Relaxing Mini-Move #5: Painting the Air (Freeing Your Arms for Action)

Susi Schropp is the busy and talented proprietor of Diva Design in New York City. When I first met Susi, she was suffering chronic neck and shoulder pain as a result of her work in print and web design, which required her to use a computer mouse almost constantly.

The mouse, invented in 1964 by computer visionary Douglas Engelbart, made possible the "graphical user interface" that is familiar to any user of a personal computer. But I'm sure Engelbart never imagined that anyone would use his epoch-making device continuously, all day long, day after day. As it turns out, even the most aptly designed mouse, when overused, can place tremendous strain on the delicate tendinous structures of the hand, wrist, and arm. And the static posture we tend to assume during prolonged mouse use can be murder on our necks, shoulders, and upper backs. Add to that the poor workstation design that is common in many industries, and you've got a recipe for disaster. (A word to the wise: Be sure to position your mouse as close to your keyboard as possible, on the same horizontal plane. Having to reach far to the side, or higher or lower than keyboard height, considerably amplifies the physical stress of using a mouse.)

For Susi, interrupting that static posture and replacing it with dynamic movement would be the key to safer, more comfortable mousing. Together we explored a wide variety of mouse-related movements, looking always for many different ways to do the same thing, ways that would engage not only Susi's fingers, hand, or wrist alone, but her entire frame. Of all these movements, one of the most helpful was also the simplest, most reflexive, and most frequently repeated.

Raising your arms to use a computer or piano keyboard, mouse, pencil, telephone, or other tool is a movement most of us do countless times in the course of a day, often without realizing that we're *doing* anything at all. Yet this seemingly innocuous movement, when poorly coordinated, can place a tremendous strain on your neck, shoulders, and back and interfere with the proper functioning of your hands and eyes.

This Mini-Move teaches you to raise and lower your arms with minimal effort and maximum freedom of movement. The secret is to precisely coordinate the movement of your arms with the movements of your hips and spine. But don't worry, you won't need to bother yourself thinking about where your hips, back, arms, and hands should be every minute of the day. Once you've got the feel of the basic arm-to-body coordination, it will all tend to happen spontaneously, without much active thought on your part. An occasional review of this Mini-Move will keep it all fresh in your mind and in your body.

Freeing your arms for action will help you to perform all of your daily activities with greater ease and comfort. As a result, you'll feel more alert and alive during your working day. You'll experience greater stamina, heightened productivity and creativity, and greater resistance to hand, wrist, back, neck, and shoulder injuries. When the workday is done, you'll find these same principles of dynamic movement will serve you well in home projects, hobbies, sports, and the arts. And when bedtime arrives, you can lay down your arms and get ready for a night of peaceful, restorative sleep.

Step 1. *Observe your sitting posture.* Find a comfortable, stationary chair, preferably one with a flat, horizontal seat. Sit on the front half of the seat, any way that you like as long as you are not leaning on the backrest.

- Take a few moments to notice how you sit. Where do you place your feet? Do you breathe freely, or do you tend to hold your breath? Do you slouch, or do you sit tall?
- Pay particular attention to your arms and hands as you sit. What part of your arms make contact with your lap? Is it your elbows? Your forearms? Your wrists or hands?
- Do you feel that your arms are in repose? Do they rest easily in your lap? Or do you feel that there is some effort required just to maintain your arms in a resting state?

Step 2. *Raise your arms.* Sit as before, on the front half of your chair. Place your right hand on your thigh near your right knee and

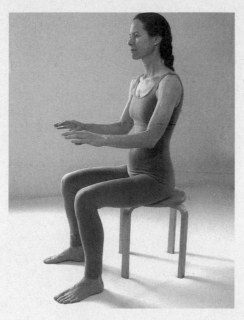

RAISE YOUR ARMS. Slowly raise both arms in front of you, as if you were reaching for your keyboard, and slowly lower your arms to your knees again.

your left hand on your thigh near your left knee. Slowly raise both arms in front of you, as if you were reaching for your keyboard, and slowly lower your arms to your knees again. Your elbows should be relaxed, not stiff, and slightly bent. Repeat this several times.

- How does it feel to raise your arms and lower them? Is it easy and comfortable, or is it a strain? Do your arms feel light and easy to manage, or do they feel heavy and cumbersome? Do you feel a strain in any other part of your body? Make a mental note of what you feel now so you can compare at the end of the exercise.

Stop and rest for a while. Continue when you are ready.

Step 3. *Raise your arms while slouching.* Sit as before, with your hands on your thighs. Now slouch a little as you learned to do in the previous Mini-Move: Incline your head forward, allow your chest to sink, round your lower back, and rock your pelvis so you

**RAISE YOUR ARMS
WHILE SLOUCHING.**
Slouch as you learned to do
in the previous Mini-Move.
Slowly raise your arms and
lower them several times in
succession. Remain slouched
the entire time as you move
your arms.

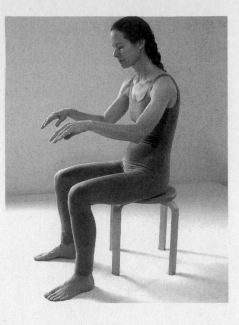

sit more on the rearward portion of your buttocks. Don't exaggerate—a gentle slouch will do.

Without recovering from this slouch, slowly raise your arms and lower them several times in succession. Remain slouched the entire time as you move your arms. At first raise your arms only an inch or so each time, gradually increasing the range with each repetition. Starting with small, slow movements allows you to detect subtle differences between one movement and the next.

- Can you feel a difference in the movement of your arms now? Does slouching like that make your arms feel lighter, or heavier? Do your arms move easily, or do they feel clumsy? Do you feel a strain in some other part of your body? Lower your arms and rest a moment.

Step 4. *Raise your arms while sitting up tall.* Slouch a little, then recover, and sit as tall as possible without strain. While holding

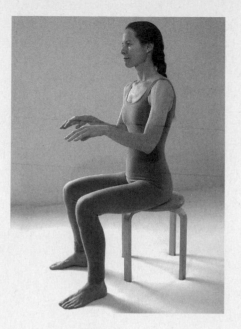

RAISE YOUR ARMS WHILE SITTING UP TALL. Sit as tall as possible without strain. While holding your body upright like that, slowly raise and lower your arms several times.

your body upright like that, slowly raise and lower your arms several times. Again, start with small movements, gradually increasing the range with each repetition. Do not slouch; remain upright as you raise and lower your arms.

- How does it feel to raise your arms now that you are sitting tall? Is it easier than when you were slouching, or not? See what you discover.

Stop and rest.

Step 5. *Synchronize your arms with your trunk.* Sit as before, on the front half of your chair with your hands on your thighs, and slouch. Slowly recover from the slouch and as you do so, slowly lift your arms. Then slowly, gradually slouch again, and slowly lower your arms. Repeat several times.

SYNCHRONIZE YOUR ARMS WITH YOUR TRUNK. Slouch. As you recover from the slouch, slowly lift your arms. Then gradually slouch again, and slowly lower your arms.

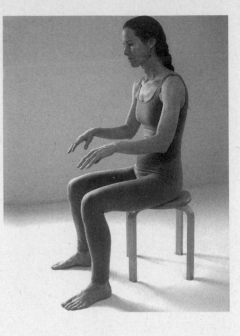

Try to synchronize the movement so that your arms and trunk go up and down at the same time. Just as you reach the lowest point of your slouch, your hands come to rest on your thighs; just as you reach your fully upright posture, your arms reach the horizontal position in front of you.

- You may find it helpful to look at your hands as they move— that will remind your head and neck to participate in the movement as well. Do many slow gentle movements like that. Rest whenever you feel the need.

You have now experimented with three variations of the movement of raising your arms: first you did it while slouching, then with your body erect, and finally with your trunk and your arms moving in concert. Which variation allowed the arms to move most freely?

Step 6. *Synchronize movement and breathing.* Sit as before, with your hands resting on your thighs. Breathe easy. As you breathe in and out, notice the gentle rising and falling of your chest.

The next time you breathe out, slouch a little, allowing your chest to sink and your back to round slightly. Then, as you inhale, recover from the slouch and sit up tall. Continue like that for several breaths until the movement becomes familiar—slouching slightly as you exhale, and recovering from the slouch as you inhale. Rest a moment.

Notice your breathing. When you find yourself naturally coming to the end of an exhalation and starting to inhale again, begin to recover from your slouch and, at the same time, slowly lift your arms. Continue raising your arms until you have completed your inhalation and are sitting tall. As you begin to exhale, gradually lower your arms and slouch again. You will find it helpful to look at your hands as they move up and down. It doesn't matter how high you lift your arms. Do what is easy and comfortable for you, and not more.

Try to synchronize your movements and breath so that you inhale, raise your arms, and sit up tall in one easy, coordinated movement. Then exhale, lower your arms, and slouch in the same way. Think that your arms are being carried up and down by the rising and falling of your chest as you breathe.

When you are learning, the quality of your movement is more important than how many movements you do, so move slowly and gradually. That allows you to pay closer attention to what you are doing with all the parts of yourself and to discover new patterns of action that are different from what you already know. Raise and lower your arms several more times. Do your arms feel lighter and easier to move than before? Rest a little.

Step 7. *Air-painting (just for fun).* Sit as before. Imagine that your forearms are paintbrushes, and your hands from the wrists

AIR-PAINTING. As you raise your arm, paint the imaginary canvas with the back of your hand in an upward-sweeping brushstroke. As you reach the top of the stroke, gently allow your wrist to bend back so that the palm side of your hand faces the canvas. Then paint the canvas with the palm of your hand in a downward-sweeping stroke.

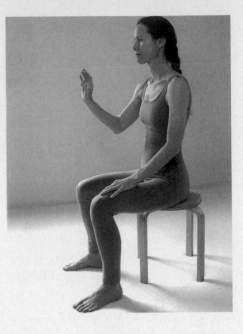

down are the long, soft, flexible bristles of the brush. The bristles have been dipped deep in wet, sloshy paint, and you are sitting in front of a huge canvas.

As you raise your right arm, paint the imaginary canvas with the back of your hand in an upward-sweeping brushstroke. As you reach the top of the stroke, gently allow your wrist to bend back so that the palm side of your hand faces the canvas. Then paint the canvas with the palm of your hand in a downward-sweeping stroke.

Repeat the movement several times. Use whatever you have learned about dynamic posture and breathing from this and the previous Mini-Move to make the movement of your arm as light, easy, and pleasurable as possible. Allow yourself to move any part of your body that helps you to paint in smooth, easy, continuous strokes.

Rest, and when you are ready to continue, repeat the movement with your left hand.

Step 8. *Advanced air-painting.* Make a complete upward and downward stroke with your right hand. Once your right hand has returned to its starting position on your thigh, raise your left hand to paint a complete upward and downward stroke. Continue painting with alternating right- and left-hand strokes for several minutes. Rest a moment.

Now paint a single upward stroke with your right hand only. As you begin to stroke downward with your right hand, raise your left hand to stroke upward. When you have raised your left hand as far as you like and your right hand has returned to its starting position, lower your left hand as you raise your right. Continue painting with overlapping right- and left-hand strokes.

- Perhaps you find yourself turning your head and eyes a little to one side and then the other to see your hands as they

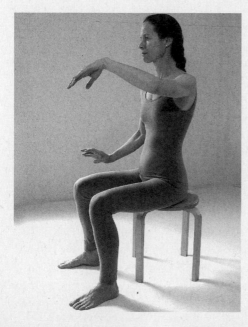

ADVANCED AIR-PAINTING. As you begin to stroke downward with your right hand, raise your left hand to stroke upward. When you have raised your left hand as far as you like and your right hand has returned to its starting position, lower your left hand as you raise your right.

move. Which hand do you look at—the one that is going up or the one that is going down?

Paint several upward and downward strokes, looking at your right hand as you raise it. As you begin to lower your right hand, gently turn your head and eyes to the left to look at your other hand as you raise it. Do several movements like that, looking at the hand that you are raising.

Try a few more movements, this time looking at the hand that you are lowering. As you lower the left hand, look at it; then gently turn your head to the other side to see the right hand as you lower it.

Which is easier, looking at the hand that goes up, or looking at the hand that goes down?

Step 9. *Put it all together.* Sit as before, on the front half of your chair. Place your right hand on your thigh near your right knee and your left hand on your thigh near your left knee. Slowly raise both arms in front of you, just as you did at the beginning of this exercise. See if it feels different now.

- How does it feel to raise your arms and lower them? Is it easier and more comfortable than before? Do your arms feel lighter and easier to manage? Notice how you are sitting on your chair. As you learn to coordinate your body movements more effectively, it becomes easier to get comfortable in your chair, and to stay that way.

Application. As you sit at your desk over the next few days, from time to time try to recall the movements you have done in this Mini-Move. Each time you raise your arms to your keyboard, remember the feeling of using your whole body to move your arms. Occasional review of the complete Mini-Move will help you make it a part of your life.

Relaxing Mini-Move #6: To Banish Neck and Shoulder Tension: Hang Loose!

Many of us accumulate tension in our necks and shoulders, especially those who work at such fixed stations as desks, computers, and control consoles. Sometimes just holding your head up all day long can feel like a tremendous effort. This simple yet powerful Mini-Move can help you relax those overtaxed muscles of the neck and shoulders. It can relieve much of the stress that comes with prolonged sitting or standing.

Here's an important bit of body wisdom: Our shoulders and arms are not part of the supporting structure of the upright body. When we're at rest, our shoulders are meant to *hang loose*. When we swing into action, our shoulders provide a stable yet mobile *anchor* for the free and spontaneous movement of our arms.

An anchor holds something in place by means of gravity. And our shoulders would make glorious anchors if we'd only let them. The problem is, many of us *lift* our shoulders continuously as we sit or stand. Instead of hanging loose, our shoulders drift upward in the direction of our ears. That's no way for an anchor to behave!

When our shoulders fail to do their job of anchoring our arms, we have to compensate in some way. To that end, we contract muscles in the arms themselves, as well as in the chest, head, neck, and back that are not really meant for that purpose. A muscle that is chronically contracted is not available to participate in movement. As a result, the free movement and expression of our arms, chest, head, neck, and back are compromised. We are quite literally "in a bind."

As you can see, this misdirected effort of the shoulder muscles throws our whole dynamic posture out of balance. It undermines the effectiveness of all the movements of the head, eyes, neck, and trunk. It wastes vital energy, inviting early fatigue. That means increased effort and strain, poor mood, and reduced pleasure in all our actions.

Why do we mis-coordinate our shoulders like this? No one really knows. It may be the result of injury or overuse, unconscious anxiety, or the residue of childhood trauma. Whatever the cause, when you can really let your shoulders hang loose, you'll heave a deep sigh of relief. That means you're on the road to self-healing. Step by step, you are approaching your goal of sounder sleep and a more peaceful life.

Step 1. *Get comfortable.* Sit upright on a chair. Place the soles of your feet on the ground. Place your hands palms down on your thighs. How does it feel to sit like that? Take a moment to notice your neck and shoulders, your back. Is there any tension? Is your breathing free and easy, or do you hold your breath?

- This Mini-Move is presented in sitting position, but it can be just as easily done in standing position, with your arms hanging at your sides, if desired. Sitting is more restful, of course.

Step 2. *Calibrate your shoulders.* Take note of the distance between the tip of your right shoulder and your right earlobe. Compare that with the distance between your left shoulder and your left earlobe. Is the distance greater on one side or the other? Try to remember what you've observed, so you can compare later.

Step 3. *Calibrate your head and eyes.* Slowly and gently turn your head and eyes to the right and to the left, without straining. Does your head turn farther to one side or the other? Which feels freer and easier, turning to the right or the left?

Now, turn your head and eyes to the right only, without force, without strain. When you are turned to the right, what part of the room can you see? Take note of some spot in the room—the corner of a chair, a clock on the wall, anything at all. You will use this as a landmark for later comparison.

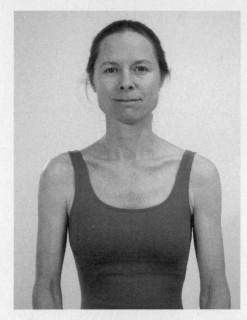

CALIBRATE YOUR SHOULDERS. Take note of the distance between the tip of your right shoulder and your right earlobe. Compare that with the distance between your left shoulder and your left earlobe.

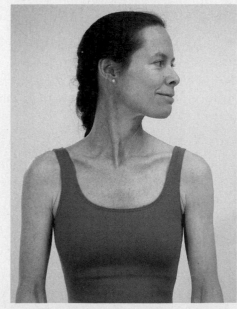

CALIBRATE YOUR HEAD AND EYES. Slowly and gently turn your head and eyes to the right and to the left, without straining. Does your head turn farther to one side or the other? Which feels freer and easier, turning to the right or the left?

Now do the same thing on the other side. Gently turn your head and eyes to the left, without straining. Choose a landmark for later comparison. Make a mental note of it.

Step 4. *Raise your right shoulder.* As you slowly inhale, gently raise your right shoulder. Just do the natural movement of raising your shoulder upward and a little toward your right ear. Now slowly exhale and gradually allow your shoulder to go back down. Repeat several times, synchronizing the movement with your breath.

RAISE YOUR RIGHT SHOULDER. As you slowly inhale, gently raise your right shoulder.

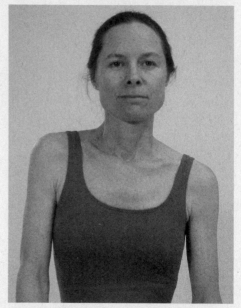

- Make the movement of your shoulder as light and easy as you can. Lift your shoulder only as high as it goes without strain. At the moment you feel that lifting the shoulder any higher would require additional effort, back off a little. You've reached the limit.
- These Mini-Moves are not like other exercises you may have learned, where faster, bigger, and harder is better. Moving

slowly and gently within the range of movement that is easy for you allows you to feel more. Your ability to feel is your most important tool for achieving greater mental and physical ease.

Step 5. *Stop, rest, and feel.* Is there any change, even a small one, of the feeling in your neck or your shoulders? Notice the distance between the tip of your right shoulder and your right ear now. Is it greater or less? Observe the difference between your right shoulder and your left. What do you feel?

Slowly turn your head to the right and to the left without strain. Which side is easier now? Does your head turn a little farther in one direction than before?

- If you're tired of sitting upright, lean back in your chair and rest a few moments. Or, lie down and take a nap if you like. You can always continue later!

Step 6. *Raise your shoulder in stages.* This time, you will raise your shoulder in three stages, synchronizing the movements with your breath. You'll be guided step by step.

Stage 1: Slowly inhale, and very gently raise your right shoulder a little bit, perhaps one-quarter of the maximum, or less. Then, keeping your shoulder where it is, slightly raised, slowly exhale. Your shoulder remains slightly raised, while you exhale fully.

Stage 2: Slowly inhale, and gently raise your shoulder another quarter of the way, or less. Then, keeping your shoulder where it is, raised about halfway or less, slowly exhale. Your shoulder remains raised, while you exhale fully.

Stage 3: Slowly inhale, and raise your shoulder a little farther. Then, keeping your shoulder where it is, raised about three quarters of the way or less, slowly exhale. Your shoulder remains raised, while you exhale fully.

RAISE THE SHOULDER IN THREE STAGES. Slowly inhale and raise your shoulder about one-quarter of the way, and hold it there. Slowly exhale. Repeat two more times, raising the shoulder higher each time. Then, slowly inhale and as you exhale, slowly lower the shoulder and relax.

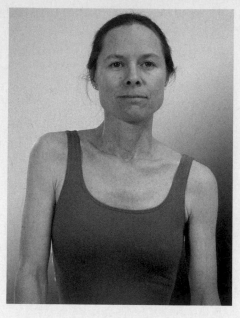

To finish: Slowly inhale and then, as you slowly exhale, gradually allow your shoulder to float all the way back down to a natural resting position. Then stop and rest for at least three complete breath cycles. Notice any apparent changes in your shoulder, neck, or back.

Repeat this sequence three to five times. Don't forget to rest after each round!

Breathe and move with minimal force. There should be nothing extreme or challenging, nothing sharp or sudden. The entire sequence should feel light, easy, and pleasurable at every step of the way.

Step 7. *Stop, rest, and feel.* Take account of the distance between your right shoulder and your right ear, and between your left shoulder and your left ear, now. Are the two distances greater or less than when you began? Does one shoulder feel more inclined to *hang loose* than the other? Which one is it?

Now, slowly turn your head and eyes to the right and left.

• Does your head turn more easily than before? Remember the landmarks you chose when we began. Can you see them? Or can you see a bit beyond them now? Is the improvement more pronounced on one side? Which side is that?

Step 8. *Raise the other shoulder.* Please repeat all the movements in Steps 4, 5, 6, and 7 with your *left* shoulder. Take all the time you need to explore the movements of the left shoulder, just as you did with the right. Do all the movements with that same slow, gentle, gradual quality. And when the instructions say to pause or rest, please do. Do not hurry!

Step 9. *Enjoy the changes in yourself.* Now that you've done this Mini-Move with both shoulders, take a few moments to observe the effects. Notice the distance between your shoulders and your ears now. Is there a little more space between them?

Slowly turn your head to the right and left and look for your landmarks in the room. Can you see past them now? Some people find that they can see the entire room behind them. It's almost like having eyes in the back of your head!

Best of all, notice how you *feel.* You may discover pleasurable physical sensations in your neck, your chest, your upper back, your arms, or anywhere you care to look. Do not be surprised if you experience a rush of pleasurable feeling in your body as your neck and shoulders "let go." If that happens, you're definitely on the right track.

Application. This Mini-Move is a perfect complement to the previous two Mini-Moves, Slouch and Recover and Air-Painting. Take the time to explore all three, and you'll achieve a more dynamic, balanced sitting posture. You'll sit and hold your head up with greater comfort and ease while using your hands and arms with greater power and precision. Believe it or not, these Mini-Moves may help you discover unexpected reserves of creative energy in yourself. Please use them for the good of all humankind. We need all the help we can get!

Chapter 4

Calm Your Mind

But you have no need to go anywhere—
Journey within yourself.
Enter a mine of rubies
    and bathe in the splendor of your own light.
                                        —RUMI

I hope you enjoyed the mindful movement experiments presented in chapter 3. If so, you now possess valuable tools you can use to relax your body and move with greater pleasure, ease, and efficiency. Instead of wasting energy on awkward, misdirected movements, you have energy to spare for creativity and self-nurturing. As a result, life is sweeter and easier, and you can enjoy it more than ever.

In this chapter we'll take another important step in our quest for sounder sleep. Here you will learn a unique type of *movement meditation* to calm your mind during waking hours. But don't worry, this kind of meditation doesn't require you to shave your head, follow a guru, or recite a mantra. You don't have to believe in any esoteric doctrine or philosophy. In fact you don't have to believe in *anything* other than the evidence of your own senses. Because when you practice these techniques, you will feel the effects immediately, the first time and every time thereafter.

Movement meditations are uniquely practical, fast-acting, easy-to-learn techniques that will bring you many of the physical and psychological benefits of traditional meditation in no time flat. Practicing these gentle movement and breathing techniques for brief periods, two or three times a day, will help you to achieve a more peaceful, balanced life. When your life is more peaceful your sleep is more peaceful. Yes, it's really that simple.

Why Daytime?

But why, you may ask, do I have to do these exercises to calm my mind during the *daytime*? I'm fine during the daytime! My problem is at night. I can't *sleep*!

The answer is that insomnia isn't just a nighttime problem. The quality and quantity of your sleep at night depends in large part on the quality of your activity during the day. For example, let's say you're one of those people, not unusual in contemporary society, who spend the whole day sprinting from one appointment to the next, juggling meetings and deadlines, and running for buses, taxis, or departing flights with nary a moment to catch your breath. It may be an exciting way to live, but it is really hard on your mind and body. You are overscheduled, overstimulated, hypervigilant, and hyperaroused. The hypothalamic-pituitary-adrenal (HPA) axis—your body's central stress response mechanism—is pumping out stress and arousal hormones, and all the systems of your body are working harder and running hotter than normal. Even when you stop to rest, your body and mind are still highly activated. You never achieve that state of quiet repose that would allow you to recover from the stress of life.

That much you probably already know. But what you may not realize is that the stress that nips at your heels during waking hours follows you right into your bedroom, undermining the quality of your nighttime sleep. I've observed this repeatedly with my clients in the business world. A fifty-five-year-old man whom I'll call Harold had suffered insomnia for several years, along with headaches and jaw pain associated with tooth grinding at night, and he was taking medication for high blood pressure. He had tried sleeping pills, too, but reported that he couldn't tolerate the side effects. For the last year, he had been "toughing it out" on three or four hours of sleep a night. He was exhausted.

Harold was the owner of a health maintenance organization with fifty employees. Amazingly, he was directly responsible for supervising the performance of each one of those employees, beginning at 6:30 a.m. each morning and ending at 9 p.m. each night, and he was quite proud of his role as a "hands-on manager." As I questioned Harold in depth about his typical day, a picture of unremitting stress began to emerge. He had people working on projects all over the country, and they relied on him for continuous input and approval. While we were together, his cell phone rang almost constantly and his pager was almost as active. He rarely stopped for lunch, and he had never considered rest breaks. He was convinced that the extreme fatigue brought on by his overwork should *promote* sleep rather than prevent it. "You work hard all day, and then you collapse into bed," was Harold's idea of normal sleep behavior.

Harold stared at me in disbelief when first I told him that being more relaxed during waking hours would help him to sleep more peacefully at night. A more peaceful life? That was the last thing on his agenda! It took some skillful negotiating on my part to get him to acknowledge that there *might* be some connection between his nonstop, high-intensity working style and his inability to sleep. But sure enough, when we started to build some movement-meditation "time-outs" into his daily routine (even prize fighters take a break between rounds, right?), Harold started to notice a difference in the quality of his life: "I'm kinder and a little more patient," he observed. More restful nights came only gradually, but Harold could feel immediately that cultivating a slightly slower and more peaceful life, with shorter working hours, was a good thing. He felt calmer and more in control. A milestone in our relationship, for me at least, was the day Harold announced that he had engaged a management consultant and was going to delegate some of his supervisory responsibilities to others who, he slyly revealed, he had been grooming for the task all along!

The sleep-impairing effects of hyperarousal have been confirmed by numerous laboratory studies. For example, a 2001 review conducted in the neurology unit of a Swiss hospital cites seven prior studies finding elevated EEG activity in the beta frequency range (12–30 cycles per second) in insomniacs during the period before sleep onset as well as during nighttime sleep. Beta activity generally indicates arousal and alertness, while quiet waking rest evokes alpha waves (8–12 cps) and peaceful sleep produces much slower oscillations in the theta and delta range (less than 4 cps). The authors identify central nervous system hyperarousal as a likely cause of insomnia. Another study from a Dayton, Ohio, veterans' hospital found increased oxygen consumption by night and day in patients with primary insomnia as compared to a control group of normal sleepers, indicating a higher metabolic rate and increased physiological activity antagonistic to natural, restful sleep. And yet another study conducted in 2004 in the Department of Psychiatry at the University of Pittsburgh analyzed stress-related changes in heart rate variability during sleep in fifty-nine healthy men and women. Participants were randomly assigned to either a speech task that was used to elicit acute stress immediately prior to sleep or a control group. Electrocardiograms (EKG) were monitored during sleep for both groups.

Results indicated a correlation between the acute induced stress and "decreased levels of parasympathetic modulation" during REM and non-REM sleep. In other words, the calming, restorative effects of sleep were blunted in the stress group.

Now some people seem to thrive on the high-stress lifestyle, at least for a time. They'll spend the whole day zooming around like Harold, and at the end they'll have dinner, relax a bit—or maybe put in a few more hours of work at home (!)—and then go right to sleep. But for many others, and probably for *you* if you're reading this book, it's not so simple. Spend the whole day in adrenal overdrive like that, and you won't be able to just turn it off at bedtime. It will take several hours for the stress hormones that have flooded your system all day to subside, allowing you to sleep. Even then, these studies indicate, your HPA axis may never quiet down enough to yield truly restful sleep.

Okay, maybe you're not the hard-driving, overachiever type described above. Maybe you're retired, or a homemaker, or lead a life of apparent leisure. It doesn't matter. You could still be living in high-stress, hyperarousal mode. For example, I have known many retired people who swear there's no stress in their lives— after all, they're *retired*! They have yet to accept that the simple fact of aging can add additional stress to our lives. Even for those in good health, their ordinary daily activities—bathing, eating and preparing food, taking care of one's home, to name just a few—take a little more time and energy. In addition, it seems that many of my retired friends have managed to become just as overscheduled, overstimulated, hypervigilant, and hyperaroused as those younger men or women clutching their briefcases, racing to catch the next flight to Cincinnati. Senior enrichment programs, social engagements, family gatherings, travel, medical appointments—all necessary and good in and of themselves—combined with inclement weather or the simple stress of *getting from here to there*, can conspire to make retired life enormously stressful. Add an illness or disability, economic uncertainty, or the loss of a spouse, and you've got all the ingredients for a stubborn case of stress-induced insomnia.

As you can see, the cause of insomnia does not reside in the bedroom alone. To paraphrase Shakespeare, "where stress lodges, sleep will never lie." That's why any comprehensive approach to insomnia must provide a way to keep those raging stress hormones at bay during waking hours. Fortunately, in most cases it doesn't take much to get your life on a more even keel. The gentle, effective Mini-Moves presented in this chapter provide you with a powerful tool you can use to that end. If you're willing to devote a little time and attention to the problem every day, you'll probably find that many, if not all, of the symptoms of hyperarousal will abate in short order. The Mini-Moves in this chapter show you how.

How will you know when you've got a handle on those pesky stress hormones? Certainly, there are medical tests you could take to measure the changes in your adrenal hormone levels as you practice the Mini-Moves, and you may want to explore that option with your doctor. But it is more likely that after a few days of practice, you will begin to feel the difference in yourself. You'll find that you feel calmer, less frazzled, and more resilient to stress during the day. And when bedtime comes, you're in just the right frame of mind and body for a delicious night of dozing and dreaming. Being more relaxed during waking hours *sets the scene* for sounder sleep.

Why Meditation?

The whole world is hurried, worried, and harried, and millions suffer as a result. We're nervous and jittery, overwhelmed and exhausted, and on top of all that, we can't sleep. There is abundant research indicating that meditation is an easy, enjoyable, no-cost solution that's right at our fingertips. Numerous studies show that meditation can be profitably practiced by almost anyone, from troubled adolescents and workers in a variety of occupations to people suffering from cancer, high blood pressure, fibromyalgia, and HIV. It has been shown to relieve anxiety, pain, stress, and depression, as well as improve mood, enhance general health, and improve sleep quality for healthy folks as well as those suffering or recovering from a wide variety of illnesses.

For example, a 2003 study conducted at the Laboratory for Affective Neuroscience at the University of Wisconsin found significant changes in brain and immune function among healthy participants in an eight-week meditation course as compared to controls. Subjects showed increased activation of the front, left side of the brain, a pattern associated with "positive affect," or good mood. After the course, both meditators and controls received an influenza vaccination. Meditators had a significant increase in antibody titers, indicating enhanced immune response as compared to controls. Interestingly, the magnitude of increase in left-sided brain activation predicted the magnitude of antibody response to the vaccine. "Meditation may change brain and immune function in positive ways," the researchers concluded.

If you run or work out, you may be interested to know of a 1995 study published in the *British Journal of Sports Medicine* that found that meditation may be a way to reduce the immunosuppressive effects of vigorous exercise. In a six-month trial, six runners who meditated following their daily workout had a significantly smaller increase in CD8+ T cells following a stress test compared to a non-meditating runner control group. Meditation, the authors conclude, may modify the suppressive influence of strenuous physical stress on the immune system. A 2000 study from the same journal reports that meditation training may aid in recovery after exercise. The study of thirty-one adult male runners found that after six months of meditation training, blood lactate concentration, an index of exercise-induced stress, was significantly decreased in the meditation group as compared to controls. You say you don't go in for running? Perhaps shooting is more to your taste: Another study found that meditation reduced tension and improved performance among a group of twenty-five elite competitive shooters.

Meditation is also good medicine when you're sick. A review of medical literature on meditation conducted at the University of South Carolina's College of Nursing in 2003 noted that "clinical effects of meditation impact a broad spectrum of physical and psychological symptoms and syndromes, including reduced anxiety, pain, and depression, enhanced mood and self-esteem, and decreased stress." The author concludes that meditation can have a positive influence on the experience of chronic illness and serve as a prevention strategy as well.

A bumper crop of recent studies attest to these findings. A 2000 University of Maryland study of non-pharmacological treatments for fibromyalgia, a chronic pain syndrome, found that a program of still and moving meditation produced significant improvement in a range of measures including sleep quality, tender points, and pain threshold. Improvement was sustained four months later. A 1993 study at a Massachusetts hospital reached similar conclusions: "a meditation-based stress reduction program is effective for patients with fibromyalgia." These findings have been borne out by the clinical experience of occupational therapist Jeanne Melvin, former program manager of Fibromyalgia and Chronic Pain Programs at Cedars-Sinai Medical Center in Los Angeles. "I use your techniques with all my patients because they are so simple and effective," she reported after taking my course.

Jeanne is presently a behavioral sleep medicine consultant to the Sleep and Autonomic Disorders Center at UCLA, and continues to use the Mini-Moves on a daily basis.

A 2004 study of the impact of stress reduction techniques on African American adolescents found that a four-month program of Transcendental Meditation produced greater decreases in systolic and diastolic blood pressure than a health education program of the same duration. This demonstrates the "beneficial impact of the TM program in youth at risk for the development of hypertension," according to the study authors.

Another 2004 study of early stage breast and prostate cancer patients, conducted in Canada, found that an eight-week mindfulness-based meditation program incorporating relaxation, meditation, gentle yoga, and daily home practice yielded significant improvement in overall quality of life, symptoms of stress, and sleep quality. Improvements in quality of life were associated with decreases in afternoon cortisol levels. The authors furthermore observed that the meditation program produced "possibly beneficial changes in hypothalamic-pituitary-adrenal (HPA) axis functioning."

Similar results were obtained in a 2004 study of organ transplant patients conducted at the University of Minnesota. A mindfulness-based relaxation course was offered 2½ hours a week for eight weeks, with a recommended 45 minutes' home practice, five days a week. The findings indicate improvement from baseline symptom scores for depression and sleep at the completion of the program. Three months later, improvement in sleep continued, and there was a significant improvement in anxiety scores, too. These results suggest that "symptom distress in transplant recipients seems to respond to mindfulness-based meditation," the authors conclude.

Another 2004 study, this one from the University of Texas,

studied the effects of a stress-reduction program including regulated breathing, meditation, and related techniques on patients with lymphoma and a control group. The meditation group reported "significantly lower sleep disturbance scores" during a three-month follow-up compared with controls. These included "better subjective sleep quality, faster sleep latency, longer sleep duration, and less use of sleep medications." We have encountered similar results with a group of ovarian cancer survivors in New York City. My associate Jae Gruenke led a four-week class emphasizing movement meditation and sleep-inducing Mini-Moves for the SHARE organization. Feedback from participants indicated considerable improvement in daytime relaxation and nighttime sleep. "Since I took the Sounder Sleep System workshop I am truly sleeping better than in many years," wrote one participant. "Incredible to believe, my sleep is deeper, and I can get back to sleep after going to the bathroom during the night. Additionally, I get up feeling well rested and refreshed from getting a good night's sleep!" As for daytime effects, this same participant reports, "I do remind myself to take a short break to practice when I'm in my office (or on the subway, bus, or taxi), to calm myself and relax. I find that when I do take these breaks, the system works very well."

What accounts for meditation's wondrous benefits? The underlying physiological mechanisms are summarized by John Ding-E Young, a physiologist and immunologist at Rockefeller University, and Eugene Taylor, a lecturer on psychiatry at Harvard, in a 1998 analysis titled "Meditation as a Voluntary Hypometabolic State of Biological Estivation." ("Estivation" is similar to hibernation, except it happens in summer instead of winter.) The authors liken the physiological state of meditation to that achieved by animals during hibernation or estivation, in which metabolism slows down (i.e., becomes hypometabolic) during periods of environmental stress or short food supply. Even the simplest meditation techniques, they observe, "appear to have persistent and measurable effects that are exactly the opposite from the fight-or-flight reflex." In the fight-or-flight response, there is a dramatic surge of adrenaline and other stress-related neurotransmitters, while "large amounts of glucose become available for quick energy metabolism, respiration rate increases, blood is shunted away from the viscera to oxygenate skeletal muscle, and the organism goes into a state of heightened vigilance." By contrast, meditation produces a hypometabolic state in which "catecholamine levels drop, galvanic skin resistance markedly increases, increased cerebral profusion is present, respiration rate . . . decreases significantly; there is also . . . lowered oxygen and CO_2 consumption, and a marked decline in blood lactate." With regular practice, they assert, "a state of internal metabolic rest becomes the baseline, rather than a constant readiness and perpetual overreaction," typical of modern life. And, note well, this is especially true for *beginning meditators,* say Young and Taylor. Of special interest to us is the authors' belief that meditation is an evolutionary survival mechanism that allows us to recover from the physical and psychological stresses of life in the modern, man-made environment.

Movement Meditation: Easy, Effective, Pleasurable

So there you have it. The verdict of modern science is, *meditation is good for you.* It can reverse the deleterious effects of stress and improve the overall quality of your life and health. If you're sick it can be a wonderful ally in your recovery process. If you have trouble sleeping, meditation alone might well improve the quality of your sleep, as several of the studies suggest. And best of all, it doesn't take years of practice to achieve positive results. Even beginners can reap immediate benefits.

Funny, isn't it, that we look to scientific studies like these to confirm for us what has been recognized by human beings on every continent for countless centuries, "since the time of Adam and Eve," some say, and which we can easily confirm with our own senses? After all, scientific theories go in and out of fashion as easily as poof skirts or Nehru jackets, but the information we glean from our own observation and experience is always fresh, accurate, and up to the moment. Even so, watching modern science play "catch up" with the wisdom of the ages is fascinating, and the findings can shed new light on human function. Furthermore, I know that some of my readers set great store in scientific evidence. But now is the time for me to set all of that aside and tell you what I have discovered, not with the tools of modern science, but by means of my own senses. It is the very special form of meditation that you're going to be learning in this chapter.

What's so special about movement meditation? Many things! The most special thing is that *you can do it.* I say that for a very specific reason, and that is that many, many people have tried meditation and "failed" at it, and therefore they believe that they are unsuited for meditation. Of course, the idea that any individual is unsuited for meditation is preposterous. That's like saying someone is unsuited for breathing or speaking or walking. Meditation reflects the innate human faculty to become deeply absorbed in thought or in the perception of an object. In doing so, we briefly withdraw our awareness from the welter of activity that constitutes our everyday world, and enter a restful, recuperative state of mind and body, free from disturbing thoughts and emotions. That gives us a valuable respite from the stress of life.

Meditation, then, in its most basic form is nothing more than focused awareness. And we are, every one of us, richly endowed with physiological and psychological mechanisms designed to make focused awareness possible. Therefore, rather than wondering whether a given individual is suitable for meditation, we need to consider whether a given form of meditation is suitable for the individual and adapt our meditation techniques accordingly. That way, each person can spontaneously find the way that works best for them. The varied movement meditations in this chapter are designed to help you do just that.

Movement meditation is easy to learn and practice. No prior experience, no special skill or aptitude is required. I have trained innumerable groups in these techniques, people from all walks of life, and the vast majority find that they work the first time, and every time after that. Of course, the first time is always special, particularly if you are discovering the peaceful inner world of meditation for the first time. You may be very surprised to find that such depths of tranquility and peace exist right there, within you. But with repeated practice, you will have even more satisfying experiences, and the calming effects will stay with you for longer and longer periods. Simply approach your movement meditation practice with sincerity, follow the instructions step by step, without hurrying, and you will succeed beyond your expectations.

Movement meditation doesn't require a big expenditure of time. You can get all the benefits by practicing two or three times a day, for ten minutes each time. (Of course you are welcome to practice longer if you wish!) Mini-Moves are exceptional in their ability to induce a state of profound repose very quickly. That is made possible by the unique structure of the Mini-Moves, which consists of alternating periods of natural body movement synchronized with breathing, alternating with periods of quiet rest. Traditional relaxation and meditation techniques require focusing the mind on an internal sound, a mental concept, or the flow of the breath. However, internal sounds, mental concepts, and the flow of the breath are rather nebulous, ephemeral phenomena—they can elude your grasp as easily as a wisp of smoke. The result is that beginning meditators often struggle to maintain their focus. Their minds wander, and pretty soon they're thinking about jobs, taxes, family responsibilities, personal health issues—and the cycle of stress resumes. As a result, they may conclude that they have failed— failed to maintain their focus, failed to relax, failed to meditate. Feeling that you have failed is extremely stressful in itself.

The movement meditation techniques presented here are designed to take the stress out of meditation. With movement meditation, you direct your attention not to a sound, a concept, or the breath, but to *gentle physical movements*. Physical movements are much easier to focus on than sounds, concepts, or breath alone, because physical movements are *concrete* and immediately present to the senses. It's easy to stay focused when you're actually *doing* something physical. The result is that instead of spending a lot of time trying to reach the meditative state—and wondering whether you're *there* yet—you will become deeply absorbed very quickly. And you'll know it! Within minutes you'll feel calmer, more peaceful, more at ease. Movement meditation produces that soothing, relaxing effect in minutes. That's why it's just right for busy people with active lives.

And best of all, movement meditation is *pleasurable*: There is no suffering involved. In our daily lives, we strive hard to achieve our goals, whatever they are. If something gets in our way, we try to overcome it by working harder, exerting greater effort. This is the "work ethic." As a result, life often feels like a struggle, a "daily grind," an "uphill battle." In movement meditation and in the sleep-inducing Mini-Moves presented in the next chapter, the soft, slow rhythm of the breath and the gentle movements of the body provide a valuable counterpoint to this effortful way of life. The movements are so light and easy, so completely free of all unnecessary effort, that they are pleasurable in and of themselves. It is simply a pleasure to move that way. With regular practice of movement meditation, some of that quality of life begins to filter into your daily life. It's a good feeling!

But, as we have seen, meditation holds more generalized benefits for the average person who isn't necessarily a seeker of higher consciousness, enlightenment, or personal liberation. Maybe that average person just wants to be a bit more relaxed, more tranquil, more mentally and emotionally stable. Maybe they want to offset some of the stress of living in a fast-paced, man-made environment. Or maybe they want to live more peacefully by day, so they sleep more peacefully at night. That is a perfectly understandable desire, and our movement meditation techniques are designed to make it not only possible, but also easy and delightful.

Because if a meditation technique is not pleasurable, what is there to make you practice it day after day? We like to eat tasty food and refreshing beverages every day; we like friendship and good company; we like satisfying work and creative endeavors; and we actively seek these things in our daily life, again and again. We all know how a well-spiced dish, cooked to perfection, stimulates the appetite and gives us pleasure, and how we look for opportunities to enjoy that dish over and over.

The same principle applies to meditation, or any other self-healing practice. If it feels good, if it's enjoyable, if it brings feelings of pleasure and peace, there is a much greater chance that you are going to pursue it with regularity. And there's no question about it, any form of meditation yields the best results when it's practiced regularly. That's why these movement meditations are pleasure oriented. Because they feel good, you'll want to practice them every day. And when you practice every day, you'll be very satisfied with the results!

Freeing Your Natural Breath

To breathe deeply, sensing how one's blood is purified through its contact with the air and how one's whole circulatory system takes on new activity and strength, this is truly an almost intoxicating delight whose aesthetic value can hardly be denied.

—JEAN-MARIE GUYAU, 1884

All of the Mini-Moves in this and the following chapter emphasize slow, easy, relaxed breathing. This natural, pleasurable way of breath, not to be confused with the forceful "deep" breathing that is widely advocated, is a key element of all our calming and relaxing Mini-Moves. Fast-paced, stressful, modern lifestyles tend to disturb all the rhythms of our lives, and this is reflected in our breath. Just as we habitually hurry from one appointment to the next, we habitually hurry from one breath to the next, too. As a result, breathing becomes fast, irregular, disorganized, effortful. When we breathe this way, we tend to feel anxious, rushed, scattered, and impatient. This is not conducive to a peaceful life or to sound sleep. And yet that is the way most of us breathe.

By contrast, light, easy, well-coordinated breathing acts on the autonomic nervous system to slow the heartbeat, reduce blood pressure, diminish muscle tone, and reduce mental activity. This produces a sense of peace and tranquility that is conducive to mental and physical ease, relaxation, and natural, restful sleep.

We are meant to breathe in accord with our ever-changing, moment-to-moment metabolic needs. Some breaths are longer, some are shorter. Some breaths are deeper, some are shallower. Left to its own devices, the body automatically calibrates each breath to ensure that we receive just the right amount of oxygen for each moment of our lives. This is the innate wisdom of the body at work.

How will you know when your breathing is truly in accord with your metabolic need? There are scientific instruments that can measure the balance of oxygen and carbon dioxide in your body very precisely, but you can't carry one of them around with you during the day. (It probably wouldn't match the decor of your bedroom, either!) Fortunately, our Creator has endowed us with some very sensitive instrumentation of our own. Whenever our breathing achieves that just right balance of oxygen and carbon dioxide that is in perfect accord with our metabolic needs, we receive an unmistakable signal from deep within ourselves. That signal is *pleasure*. In that moment, when the respiratory movements of our bodies are perfectly matched to our metabolic needs, the simple act of breathing in and out is exquisitely pleasurable. Let pleasure be your guide, and you will be well on your way to freeing your natural breath.

When we are relaxing or falling asleep, our consumption of oxygen declines precipitously. The metabolic need for oxygen is much less than when we're sitting at a desk, giving a speech, or running to catch a train. The more active and alert we are, the faster is our heart rate, the higher is our blood pressure, and the more oxygen we expend. As we relax, our heart rate slows, our blood pressure declines, and our oxygen consumption declines significantly. By the time we've entered the early stages of sleep, oxygen consumption is typically 13 to 15 percent less than during quiet waking rest.

Curious, isn't it, then, that so many relaxation techniques encourage voluntary deep breathing? Because for our purposes, for the purposes of relaxation and restful sleep, we require less oxygen, not more. In my experience and observation, if we can just let the breath alone, without trying to control it, the body will take just as much oxygen as it needs, no more, no less. Moreover, voluntary breathing may activate areas of the brain that are associated with arousal, rather than rest and relaxation. Consider the following two studies. One, a Danish study of regional cerebral blood flow (rCBF) during light sleep, found decreased blood flow to the premotor cortex and cerebellum, indicating "a decline in preparedness for goal directed action during stage-1 sleep." Yet an earlier study performed in England found that volitional breathing *increased* rCBF to these very same areas of the brain. In other words, mucking about with your breathing is more likely to wake you up than it is to put you to sleep. Just let your breathing take its own course, and sleep will come to you sweetly, in its own good time.

Consider also the findings of Australian researchers Gradisar and Lack, who studied the relationship between sleep initiation and body temperature regulation. They discovered that no matter what time of day sleep is initiated, there is a rapid increase in finger temperature (1–3 degrees Celsius) beginning three hours prior to the onset of sleep, and that this change seems to trigger other, subsequent shifts in core body temperature, next in subjective sleepiness, and finally in objective sleepiness as measured by EEG. But several studies have identified a phenomenon called the "inspiratory gasp response" (IGR), in which voluntary deep breathing activates sympathetic nerve pathways to constrict the blood vessels in the skin, especially the skin of the hands. Generally speaking, anything that activates the sympathetic nervous system tends to wake you up, and anything that constricts blood vessels of the fingers will make your hands colder, not warmer. So it may be that repetitive, voluntary deep breathing interferes with one of the key physiological triggers of the sleep process. By contrast, the calming Mini-Moves in this chapter will very often produce a significant increase in finger temperature, which you will very plainly feel—yet another way in which they set the stage for sounder sleep.

Consider also an experiment I did in my own practice a few years ago. For one month I asked every new student who came into my office to simply "take a deep breath," while I observed what happened. (This was inspired by an illustration in Ida Rolf's book, *Rolfing*.) Each one did something unique, but almost all, with very few exceptions, made a tremendous effort. Some powerfully hoisted their chests, others collapsed their chest. Some violently puffed out their bellies, others sucked them in. Some hiked up their shoulders, others threw them back, military fashion. All in all, it was a symphony of misdirected effort. The impression was of strain, and in some cases, outright pain. Clearly, this was not the breath of peace and tranquility. This was not the breath that would facilitate an easy, gentle slide into sleep.

If this is what people do when you ask them to take a deep breath, what can our physical educators and therapists be thinking when they urge people to practice "deep abdominal breathing"? I once gave a presentation for a large group of patients at a hospital in the Los Angeles area. After I had guided the crowd through one of my natural breathing techniques, I took questions. An older lady recounted her long struggle with chronic obstructive pulmonary disease (COPD). I had noticed her as I circulated around the room during the breathing lesson. When we began, she had been remarkable for her grayish pallor. By the end of the segment, she had "pinked up" rather nicely, and her face bore a serene expression.

"My doctor has instructed me to do 'deep abdominal breathing,'" she said, eyes wide as saucers, spreading her arms to indicate the prescribed volume of breath, "but this is something *quite* different!"

"How so?" I asked, uncertain of her meaning.

"Well," she continued, "when I try to do the deep breathing, I feel like I'm suffocating. I'm trying to gobble up air, but I can never get enough. But what you've just taught us feels *wonderful*! Do you think it's okay? Am I getting enough air?"

I told her that I thought she was, but that of course she must have a talk with her doctor and ask whether he or she would like her to continue the deep breathing or to explore the alternative I had offered her. With her doctor's advice, she would certainly be able to make up her own mind.

Full Breathing or Deep Breathing?

Rather than deep breathing, I advocate "full breathing." What does it mean to breathe fully? To answer that, we must first ask what it means to breathe. Breathing is movement. In order to breathe in, we mobilize our diaphragm, which is the principal muscle of respiration, as well as, to a varying extent, the muscles of our neck, shoulders, chest, and abdomen. These muscular contractions not only cause the lungs to draw in air, but they also act on the skeleton, the mechanical armature of the body. As we inhale, the ribs rise and expand, and the spine lengthens and extends. As we exhale, the chest sinks and the spine flexes and shortens. (This is not the only possible pattern, but it is a general description of a typical one.) Each breath mobilizes the skeleton, producing a pulsation that ripples from head to toe through the entire frame. This gentle, ever-changing, ever-present pulsation nourishes and nurtures us, bringing oxygenated blood, pleasurable movement, and the welcome sensation of aliveness to every cell in our bodies. And each breath, each of these full-bodied pulsations, is as unique and different as one snowflake is from another, each is custom tailored to meet our momentary metabolic need. Breathing is the primal pulsation of life. This is the essence of our vitality and the life force that sustains us.

If any part of the body is chronically contracted, frozen, or otherwise unable to surrender to this gentle, all-encompassing pulsation, however, then our breath and indeed our vitality itself are constrained and compromised. Don't take my word for it! You can easily confirm this for yourself. Sit or lie quietly and allow your breathing to flow in and out several times, without any special effort. Don't hurry. Relax your lips and tongue, your eyes, your brow. Now, notice which parts of yourself move as you breathe, and how much: your chest, your belly, your back, neck and shoulders, and any other part of your body. How does it feel to breathe and move like that? Is it easy, or not? Is it pleasurable, or not? Is it satisfying, or not? Do you feel really alive, or do you feel something else?

Now, form your mouth into a frown and hold it. Continue breathing, again without any special effort, and feel the difference. What parts of your body move as you breathe, and how much now? How does it feel to breathe now? Is it easy, or not? Is it pleasurable, or not? Is it satisfying, or not? Do you feel really alive or do you feel something else? And which do you prefer, the feeling of breathing with your lips relaxed or the feeling of breathing with your lips contracted in a frown? Can you feel that the contraction of the muscles of your frowning mouth interferes with your breath and undermines your pleasure and vitality? Can you imagine how it would affect the quality of your life if you had the habit of frowning all the time? Sadly, some people do!

Now here's the antidote: Continue breathing without effort, but now, each time you inhale, softly smile, as if you're savoring a pleasant memory or meeting a beloved friend. Each time you exhale, relax your lips completely. How does it feel to breathe now, with a smile playing across your lips? Try it, and see what you discover.

Now you know a little something about what it means to breathe, at least from my personal point of view. What, then, does it mean to breathe *fully*? Breathing fully means that *every part of your body is available to participate in the movements of respiration.* That doesn't mean that every part of your body *will* participate in every breath. That is an unrealistic ideal. But it does mean that every part is *available* to participate when the need arises. When you breathe fully, your breath can continuously adapt itself to your moment-to-moment, ever-changing metabolic needs. How can you achieve full breathing? Simply allow your breathing to be light, easy, and natural. Interfere as little as possible. Just let it be. That's the way to free your natural breath.

Paradoxically, many people find themselves unable to achieve this sort of natural, uninflected breathing unassisted. Their habitual breath is fast, choppy, and irregular, or otherwise disturbed and disorganized. For some, the agonized activity that is their breath has become quite unconscious. And the moment their breath becomes an object of their attention, it is subject to some other distortion. Some huff and puff, some forcefully expel the air through pursed lips, some habitually slow the air by contracting the muscles of the nose and throat, as is taught in some forms of yoga.

Clearly, help and guidance are required to allow the natural breath to emerge. To this end, I have developed some very gentle, pleasurable Mini-Moves meant to help people achieve light, easy breathing that is fully in accord with our moment-to-moment metabolic needs. Sidestepping the kind of forceful, mis-coordinated efforts usually associated with voluntary "deep" breathing, these Mini-Moves enable you to free your natural breath effortlessly. Two examples are presented in this chapter: "L.E.S.S. Is More," and "Making Room." I have seen wondrous results with many, many people, whether healthy or ill, from all walks of life. Once the natural breath asserts itself, there is an immediate increase in vitality and pleasure. Try it, and see for yourself!

Breathing and Movement: Natural Partners

Breathing and movement are natural partners in the process of self-nurturing and self-healing. The reason is that breathing *is* movement. Without movement, breathing is unthinkable. And the movements of respiration, that is, the many varied movements that your body does in order to breathe, are the most essential, the most familiar, the most *vital* movements of all. Because whether you are aware of it or not, you are doing those movements all the time, from the very first moment of your birth, even when you're asleep or under deep anesthesia. Even *before* the moment of your birth, your mother's body made those same movements, and you felt them and listened to them and were moved by them. They are truly one of the fundamental rhythms of life.

They're also the easiest, safest, and the most effortless movements you can make. You could go to the gym or a yoga class and do all sorts of vigorous exercises, and sooner or later, no matter how gifted you are, you'll give yourself a stiff neck or a sore back or some sort of ache or pain. But the movements of respiration, if you just let them be as nature meant them to be, will never give you anything but ease and pleasure. They're perfectly familiar to the body and completely wholesome in every way—they are the "mother's milk" of movement. As a result, the movements of respiration have a very special quality that can be relied upon at any time for self-comforting, self-nurturing, and self-healing.

Principles of Natural Breath

What follows is a list of general principles of natural breathing. Don't worry, you needn't commit them to memory! You will find these principles repeated again and again in the Mini-Moves that follow.

1. Make no effort to breathe deeply, or any special way. Make no effort at all. Breathing should be, quite literally, the easiest thing in the world.

2. Simply allow the breath to come and go of its own accord. When you inhale, simply allow the breath to arrive. When you exhale, just let it flow out.

3. Let your breathing be Light, Easy, Soft, and Slow. The letters L-E-S-S spell less. When it comes to breathing for rest, relaxation, and sleep, less is more.

4. Take all the time you need for each breath. That means, take all the time you need for each out-breath; take all the time you need for each in-breath; take all the time you need between each out-breath and the subsequent in-breath.

5. Breathe *fully* rather than *deeply*. Full breathing means that all parts of your body are available to participate in the movements of respiration. The gentle Mini-Moves will help you to achieve full breathing without any effort on your part.

6. Don't gulp, gasp, or grab air. When you are deeply relaxed, your need for oxygen is less than when you're active. Whether you're in action or in repose, breathe fully, and you automatically receive exactly the right amount of oxygen for each moment of your life.

7. When you are getting the right amount of oxygen, you'll feel pleasure. The simple act of breathing in and breathing out becomes exquisitely pleasurable. That is your ever-present reminder of the joy of being alive!

Achieving a More Balanced Life

Occasionally someone asks me if these movement meditation techniques are not an escape from reality. On the contrary, I answer, they are a way of getting in touch with the *totality* of reality. You see, there is an outer reality that is happening all around you, and there is an inner reality that is happening inside of you. The outer reality is the physical world, and the inner reality is the spirit, or the soul. In our culture, we tend to focus on the outer reality almost exclusively, and we tend to forget, ignore, or deny the inner reality most of the time except in certain ritualized circumstances.

To forget, ignore, or deny the inner reality, the spirit or soul, is not a balanced way to live. It saps our energy and dampens our spirit. It's as if you went to work and just stayed there endlessly, without ever coming home to rest. That would be very stressful, and you'd be completely burned out in no time.

The same goes for our minds. We attune our minds to the outer reality so we can play an active role in the world around us. We use our minds to work and play; to think, speak, and express ourselves; to interact with other people. However, it is equally important that we attune our minds to the inner reality so we can rest, meditate, contemplate, and reflect on our actions. This is our inner source of spiritual nourishment, moral and aesthetic perception, and creative insight and inspiration.

This inner reality, when we know how to utilize it for our own benefit, is our personal resource for peace, tranquility, and rest. Lingering there in a state of purposeful inaction, we can forget the clock, forget the telephone, forget the computer; we can forget all the monstrous machines to which we have surrendered our destinies. For that moment, we suspend our ceaseless *do*ing, and we experience what it means to just *be*, unburdened by the stresses and strains of daily life. It's like coming home to your self.

And then we confront a curious fact: We are so strongly identified with what we *do,* that when we stop doing to simply *be,* we may not even recognize ourselves! When we're in that state, our thoughts, our emotions, our very bodies are so different from what we've become accustomed to, it's as if we're strangers to ourselves. But it doesn't take long for the realization to dawn on us: This is the way I was, once, a long time ago. This is me, unencumbered by the stresses and strains of daily life.

It is wonderful to discover that this kinder, gentler, more relaxed image of ourselves is still present, there, inside us. We'll want to take some time to reacquaint ourselves with this softer side of our self-image. This is a process of self-nurturing and self-realization. This is a process of self-healing. Once you've embarked on the path of self-healing, even though you may prefer to proceed very slowly and gradually, you will find that you're able to resume your outer-directed actions with renewed vigor and enthusiasm. After that brief break in the action, your mind will be sharper than ever. And you really must take a look in the mirror, for you will almost certainly see a happier, healthier, more energetic person there.

Some Thoughts on Eyes

Three of the Mini-Moves in this chapter employ eye movements for a calming effect. The first one is called "Things Are Looking Up!" That Mini-Move has its own unique calming effect, and it will also help you to get very comfortable with gentle upward movements of the eyes, eyelids, and brow that you'll encounter again later in the chapter, in the "Main Squeeze" and a "Twist of the Wrists." Why all these eye movements, and why do they all go upward but never down or to the sides? I'm glad you asked!

You're probably aware that when a person faints, all his muscles go limp and his eyes roll upward, as if he were looking up. That's why we see the whites of his eyes. You may not know that the same thing happens when you relax very, very deeply. The reason has to do with the architecture of the eyeball: Its center of gravity is not the same as its axis of rotation, rendering it slightly lop-sided, with the greater mass behind the axis. That means that when you're awake, you must continuously activate the eye muscles to bring the front of the eyeball down to meet the horizon so you can see what's going on around you. When you relax deeply, you cease that effort, and your eyes roll up.

Bringing your eyes down to the horizon allows you to see what's in front of you, but it's important for another reason as well. In addition to vision, your eyes also have an *orienting* func-tion. In order to maintain the integrity of your experience and action, your brain needs to know the position of your body in space at all times. To this end, your eyes continuously scan your environment, sending the information they gather to the brain. The brain uses this information to create a coherent map of the body and its position in surrounding space. This map is revised on a moment-to-moment basis. That's one reason why an Olym-pic diver can jump off a diving board, execute a series of complex gymnastic maneuvers in midair, and still enter the water in perfect vertical alignment. That's orientation!

This orienting function of the eyes is an essential component of normal waking consciousness. But when you roll your eyes up, orienting temporarily ceases, and the brain stops receiving the visual signals that tell it where the body is in space. As a result, normal waking consciousness is interrupted and your brain shifts into an "altered state," which simply means that for as long as you choose, you will see, hear, think, and feel differently than usual. In the particular state evoked by rolling your eyes, my experience and observation indicate that the volume of your thoughts tends to become considerably reduced and your mind becomes very still. Or, as a chronic-pain patient reported, "When I roll my eyes like that, I can't keep a thought in my head!"

If you are one of the millions plagued by obsessive, repetitive, self-defeating, or anxiety-producing thoughts, that ability to use eye movements to *slow your thoughts* can be a real godsend. It will calm your mind and give you a brief respite from the stress of life. For those few moments, whatever you're holding on to, you can just let it go. As a result, you may find yourself breathing a deeply pleasurable sigh of relief as your fear, your anxiety, and all your unrealistic expectations start to lose their grip on you. And you can achieve all that without potions or pills!

A final note on the eyes and sleep. Many sleep researchers have observed that in the early stages of sleep, our eyes involuntarily make slow, rhythmic, vertical rolling motions. Why? I haven't been able to find an explanation. But I suspect it works something like this: The transition from waking to sleep is not a one-way street—we drift from Stage 1 into Stage 2 and back again several times before finally and decisively drifting off to sleep. As long as you are in Stage 1, the lightest stage of sleep, your mind and body are still aroused enough to bring the eyes down to the horizon, a hallmark of the waking state. Each time you drift into Stage 2, arousal peters out, your muscles lose their tone, and your eyes drift upward. Each time you return to Stage 1, your eyes come back down. Now, here's a brain teaser for you. As we fall asleep we involuntarily do slow, rhythmic, upward-rolling movements of the eyes. Can it be that by *intentionally* doing slow, rhythmic, upward-rolling eye movements, we can actually usher ourselves in the direction of slumber? In "Things Are Looking Up," you'll try it yourself. See what you discover!

Your Daily Practice of the Calming Mini-Moves

These Calming Mini-Moves are a perfect fit for your busy lifestyle. You can do them anytime, anywhere (except, of course, while you're driving or operating heavy machinery!). That's a good thing, because the Mini-Moves have a cumulative effect. The more you practice, the better the results. But let's not set up any unrealistic expectations. If you can take ten minutes, or more, out of your busy day, *today*, and do one of these relaxing Mini-Moves, you will begin to feel better already. Good for you! That in itself is a great success.

Now consider this: If you could set aside those same ten minutes, or more, every day, and stick to it, you would be laying the foundation for lasting serenity and greater peace of mind. Just the act of doing that one positive, self-nurturing thing for yourself every day builds up a positive momentum that will lift your spirits day by day. You'll have more energy, feel more joy, and be more at peace with yourself and others.

After a while, it might be that you will really start to look forward to that daily encounter with peace and tranquility. And it might be that you really enjoy it and you start to see some positive changes in your life as a result: calmer, more peaceful, happier. Then, and only then, you are welcome to up the ante to ten minutes or more, two or even three times a day. Make that modest commitment, and you will be well along the path to self-healing. And when you start practicing the Lulling Mini-Moves in chapter 5, you'll get the very best possible results.

Calming Mini-Move #1: L.E.S.S. Is More
(For Deep Relaxation, Breathe Fully Rather than Deeply)

Less and less do you need to force things
until finally you arrive at non-action.
When nothing is done,
nothing is left undone.

—TAO TE CHING, *Stephen Mitchell, trans.*

Proper breathing is essential for relaxation and sounder sleep. But what is proper breathing? There's a very simple answer. For our purposes—for the purposes of relaxation and sounder sleep—proper breathing is L.E.S.S.: light, easy, soft, and slow.

Light means you can breathe without force. You neither draw your breath in nor push it out. Just allow it to come and go of its own accord.

Easy means you can breathe without effort. You are by nature a living, breathing being. In order to breathe, you don't have to *do* anything. Just *be*.

Soft means that your breath is gentle and continuous. Everything happens gradually—no need to huff or puff.

Slow means you can breathe without hurrying. Simply take all the time you need for each breath.

Therefore, when it comes to breathing, L.E.S.S. is more. More natural, more pleasurable, more peaceful. This is one of the fundamental secrets of sounder sleep.

Happily, every one of us can achieve light, easy, soft, slow breathing quite easily. That's right. No exotic, complicated practices are required. In fact, you may find that once you have tried this approach to breathing, it seems rather familiar. That's because it's not too very different from the way you already breathe. It's just a little lighter and easier, a little softer and slower. And it feels very, very good.

If you feel like yawning, or breathing a sigh of relief right about now, be my guest! There you go.

The gentle, step-by-step techniques that follow are designed to help you achieve light, easy, soft, and slow breathing in the simplest, most practical way possible. Just follow my spoken instructions, keep an open mind, and give yourself permission to enjoy each step in the process. Always remember, enjoyment is your key to greater self-awareness and self-healing.

Step 1. *Get ready.* Please lie down on your back on the floor or in bed. If you need pillows or a blanket, please get them now. Make yourself as comfortable as possible.

Step 2. *Observe yourself at rest.* Rest quietly for a time and see how it feels to lie like that. Are you at ease, or do you feel tense and restless? You needn't change anything. Just see what is.

Now, simply notice how you breathe. Does your breathing feel easy and natural? Or do you make some effort to breathe in a particular way?

- Throughout this program, just breathe in the way that comes most naturally to you, without trying to control your breath in any way. Any changes in your breath will occur spontaneously, without any effort on your part.
- To inhale, you don't have to do anything. Just allow the breath to arrive. Your body automatically supplies itself with just the right amount of oxygen for this moment.
- To exhale, just allow the breath to flow out. Exhaling doesn't require any effort at all. Simply let your body be at ease, and the air flows out.
- Make no effort to breathe deeply, or any other way. Intentional deep breathing can create a feeling of strain or effort. As a result, deep breathing may produce more stress than it

relieves. Light, easy breathing is effortless. It counteracts the effects of stress. It brings you pleasure and peace.

- Do not hurry. Take all the time you need for each breath. Taking time is one of the fundamental principles of light, easy breathing.

Step 3. *Explore the lower breathing space.* Now place your hands side by side, palms down, on your lower abdomen. Gently spread your thumbs apart from the rest of your hands. If possible, arrange your hands so that the tips of your thumbs touch each other just above your navel, and the tips of your index fingers also touch each other below your navel. The space between your hands forms a triangular or heart-shaped opening.

EXPLORE THE LOWER BREATHING SPACE. Place your hands side by side, palms down, on your lower abdomen.

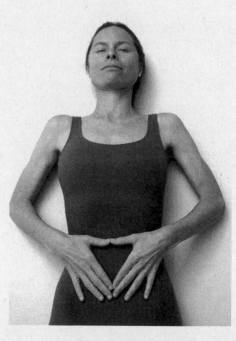

- It is most important that you make yourself completely comfortable in this position. If when you position your hands as instructed, your elbows do not reach the ground, please place a pillow or folded towel under each elbow. That will allow you to relax your arms.

Continue breathing naturally and observe what happens. As you inhale, your belly rises and expands. Since your hands are resting on your belly, your hands rise, too. Then, when you exhale, your belly falls, and your hands fall with it.

- Your hands are very sensitive. Holding your hands on your belly makes it easy to feel how your body moves as you breathe.

As you continue breathing like that, you will notice a curious thing. Each time you inhale and your belly swells and rises, the contact between your thumbs and between your index fingers becomes lighter and less distinct. You may even feel the thumbs or index fingers breaking contact and moving apart.

Each time you exhale, and your belly sinks, the tips of your thumbs and the tips of your index fingers move back together again.

- Do not move your hands intentionally. Just allow them to be carried up and down, together and apart, by the rising and falling of your belly. Your breath does the movement, not you.

Continue breathing like that for a few minutes, and just observe. You inhale, and your fingers move apart. You exhale, and your fingers move together again.

- Remember, make no effort to breathe deeply. Make no effort to breathe any special way. Let the innate wisdom of your own mind and body determine how you will respond to this gentle experiment in natural breathing.

Step 4. *Rest and observe your breath.* Allow your hands and arms to lie comfortably at your sides. Rest quietly and feel the result of what you have done. You may discover that without any effort on your part, without any trying, there has been a change, perhaps subtle, perhaps less so, in the way you breathe.

Perhaps you notice that your belly is a little freer to move with the rising and falling of your breath, and that your breathing seems a little lighter, a little easier than before.

You may feel that your breathing is a little slower. Remember, "slower" simply means unhurried. Make no effort to breathe slowly. Simply take all the time you need for each breath.

You may notice that the movements of your body as you breathe feel a little *softer*. If so, you're definitely on the right track.

Or you may feel *nothing in particular* at this moment. If so, you needn't be concerned. Some of us may take a little longer to feel the effects of these subtle explorations. Simply continue to follow these step-by-step instructions in your own way, at your own pace, and you will get all the benefits.

Step 5. *Explore the middle breathing space.* Now, with the tips of your fingers, find your lowermost ribs on either side of your body. Find the descending curve of the lower ribs by touching there with your fingertips. Your lowermost ribs form the boundary between your chest and your belly.

Place your right hand on the lowermost rib on the right, palm down, so that the rib is cradled in the crease of the palm of your hand. Your right thumb rests on your chest, above the lowermost

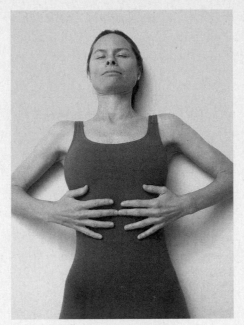

EXPLORE THE MIDDLE BREATHING SPACE. Place your right hand on the lowermost rib on the right, palm down, so that the rib is cradled in the crease of the palm of your hand. Place your left hand in the same position on the left side.

rib, and the other four fingers rest below the rib, on your belly. Place your left hand in the same position on the left side.

You may be able to arrange your hands so that the tips of your middle and index fingers touch each other. Or simply place your hands on your ribs wherever it's most comfortable for you. You can just imagine that your fingertips are touching, and you will get all the benefits. Look for the place where your hands just seem to fall into place, like the handset of a telephone resting on its receiver. Just right.

With your hands cradling your lower ribs like that, simply breathe easily and notice what happens. Just as your lower abdomen has its own characteristic rising and falling movement, so do your ribs. Breathing doesn't just happen in your lungs; your whole torso moves in order to direct the air in and out of your body.

As you inhale, your ribs expand and rise upward. The contact between your fingers gets lighter, and your fingers may move apart slightly. As you exhale, your ribs sink, and your fingers move back together again.

- Your hands are very sensitive. Holding your hands on your ribs makes it easier to feel how your body moves as you breathe. The changes in the contact of the fingers help you feel the movement more easily.
- This doesn't require a lot of thought. Instead, just allow yourself to feel—this breath, this movement, this moment. When thinking is replaced by feeling, your mind becomes very still and your whole body relaxes. Whatever your mind is holding on to, you can just let it go.

Continue breathing like that for several minutes, and observe the rising and falling of your lower ribs and the changes in the quality of the contact between your fingers. You inhale, and your fingers move apart. You exhale, and your fingers move together again.

- Again, make no effort to breathe deeply. Make no effort to breathe any special way. Let the innate wisdom of your own mind and body determine how you will respond to this experience of natural breathing.

Step 6. *Rest and observe your breath.* Allow your hands and arms to rest at your sides. Rest quietly and feel the result of what you have done. You may discover that without any voluntary effort on your part, there has been a noticeable change in the way you breathe. You may feel that your ribs move more freely with the rising and falling of your breath, and that your breathing seems a little lighter, a little easier than before. Maybe it's a little slower, a little softer.

- The amount of oxygen your body needs changes from moment to moment depending on what you're doing and how you feel. When your breathing is light and easy, you automatically receive just the right amount of oxygen for action or repose, for waking, or for sleep at each moment of the day and night.
- Notice how it feels to breathe that way. You may discover that the simple act of breathing in and breathing out is very pleasurable, all by itself. You may notice those pleasurable feelings somewhere in your chest or your belly, in your neck, back or shoulders, or anywhere in your body, as you softly breathe in and breathe out. Because your body's needs are being met with such exquisite accuracy, you will tend to feel a sense of profound well-being and inner peace.
- When you can feel that the simple act of breathing in and breathing out is a pleasure, then you are in touch with the joy of being alive. That feeling of joy is always right there, inside of you, in every moment of your life. All you have to do is breathe, and feel.

Step 7. *Explore the upper breathing space.* Now, bring your hands to the upper part of your chest, below your collarbones and above your breast. Arrange your hands so that the tips of your middle fingers lightly touch each other in the middle of your chest. Or, simply place your hands on the upper part of your chest wherever it's most comfortable for you. You can just imagine that your fingertips are touching, and you will get all the benefits.

**EXPLORE THE UPPER
BREATHING SPACE.** Bring
your hands to the upper part
of your chest, below your
collarbones and above your
breast. Arrange your hands
so that the tips of your
middle fingers lightly touch
each other in the middle of
your chest.

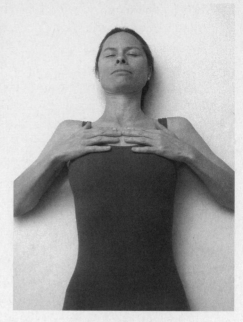

Again, make sure you're comfortable in this position. Place a
pillow or folded towel under your elbows if needed.

As you inhale, can you feel that your chest gently rises under
your hands? You may notice the tips of your middle fingers moving apart just a little bit as your chest rises. As you exhale, can you
feel how your chest gently falls? The tips of your fingers move
back together as your chest falls.

- As before, holding your hands on your chest makes it a little
  easier to feel how your chest moves as you breathe. You are
  using your hands as a biofeedback system.
- Breathing is a natural process. And like all natural processes,
  it may be somewhat irregular. You may breathe a little faster,
  a little slower. You may breathe a little deeper, or a little shal-

lower. There may be occasional lulls, when your breath becomes very still for a time. It doesn't matter, as long as your breathing is light, easy, soft, and slow.

- Remember, the letters L.E.S.S., "less," stand for light, easy, soft, and slow. When it comes to breathing, L.E.S.S. is more. More natural, more pleasurable, more peaceful.

As your chest rises and falls, continue to follow the subtle changes in the contact between your middle fingers. That simple sensory feedback mechanism is literally right at your fingertips, any time of the night or day. Just rest quietly and follow the movements of your breath. You don't have to lift a finger.

Continue resting quietly, enjoying that slow, soft quality of breath. You may keep your hands where they are, or rest them anyplace you choose. Notice how easy and light the movements of your chest are as you effortlessly inhale and exhale. When your body is free to move with your breath, your breath becomes fuller and freer without any additional effort on your part.

The whole world may be hurried, worried, and harried. You don't have to be. When you allow yourself to take all the time you need for each breath, the simple act of breathing in and breathing out is a pleasure. The past is over and done, and the future has yet to be. In this moment, in this breath, life is beautiful. It brings you pleasure and peace.

Practice these simple, natural breathing techniques first thing in the morning, and you will start your day with a peaceful feeling. At midday, they provide a welcome antidote to the stress of life. And at bedtime, they'll help you become deeply relaxed and receptive to those waves of sweet fatigue that draw you irresistibly toward rest and repose, so the warm luxury of slumber will come to enfold you. And soon enough, you will lie warm in the gold of dawn.

Calming Mini-Move #2: Making Room (For Fuller, Freer Breathing)

Here's another technique you can use to recover your natural breathing rhythm, this time in the side-lying position. If you have done the Relaxing Mini-Move "Lengthening One Side" in chapter 3, you are already familiar with the movements addressed in this Calming Mini-Move. Here, you will discover that those same movements that you learned occur automatically, without any voluntary action on your part, when you breathe. Whenever you tune in to those subtle pulsating movements of the breath, you become very calm and tranquil. In chapter 5, we'll employ some of these same movements in a very effective sleep-inducing Mini-Move, the Ziggurat. Stay tuned!

I have found another application for this particular Mini-Move. A couple of years ago I was on a surfing trip. As I walked toward shore in the shallows, I got caught by a rogue wave. It lifted me up, turned me over, then slammed me down on the sand. No big deal—surfers take this kind of abuse all the time—but we usually expect to be pretty sore afterward. But this time, I found myself a pillow and a quiet spot on the beach, and I lay there for half an hour just "Making Room." The next day, I felt just fine, I was back in the surf! I have tested this technique again and again after many kinds of physical trauma. I've taught it to people with occasional aches and pains, as well as those with chronic pain, and they all love it. Of course, it's not a cure-all, but it seems to have the wonderful ability to soothe and to heal. Try it, and see what you discover.

Step 1. *Starting position.* Lie on your right side on a bed or on a mat or carpet on the floor. Place a pillow under your head for support. (If for any reason you're not comfortable lying on your right side, lie on your left side. You can easily reverse all the instructions.)

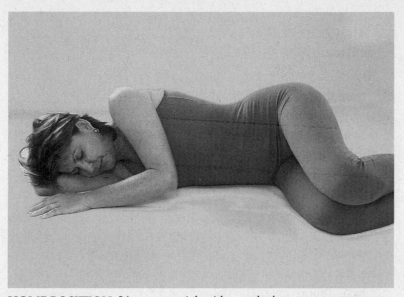

HOME POSITION. Lie on your right side on a bed or on a mat or carpet on the floor.

Bend your knees and hips comfortably so that your knees lie more or less in front of you. Your left leg lies on top of your right. Place your arms in any position that's comfortable for you. You may want to place a pillow or a folded blanket between your knees for greater comfort.

Step 2. *Observe yourself in repose.* Notice how your body makes contact with the surface it is lying on. Which part of your head presses against the pillow most distinctly? Is it your temple, your ear, your cheek, your jaw?

Notice how the side of your neck makes contact with the pillow. Does your neck feel like it is well supported by the pillow?

How about your right shoulder? Does it press forcefully into the bed or mat you're lying on, or is it supported softly, evenly, comfortably? Please make any adjustments needed for your own comfort.

Notice your ribs on the right side, your right hip, your right leg, knee, ankle, foot. Just feel how each part of yourself is supported by the earth beneath you.

Step 3. *Rest and breathe.* Rest quietly for a time and let your breathing be easy and natural. Make no effort to breathe deeply, or any special way. As you continue to rest and breathe, simply *take all the time you need for each breath.*

That means, take all the time you need for each in-breath. Take all the time you need for each out-breath. Take all the time you need *between* each in-breath and out-breath.

- Taking all the time you need doesn't require you to *do* anything. It just means, there's no need to hurry! When your breathing becomes truly unhurried, so will you. Your body will begin to relax, and your mind will become clear and calm.

Step 4. *Observe the movements of the breath.* As you rest quietly like that, breathing easily, simply notice whether any part of your body *moves* as you *breathe.* Look for the *physical sensation* of movement.

- Breathing is movement. Even when we are lying very still, our bodies are in motion, moving oxygen in and out of our lungs. And like all of our movements, the movements of the breath produce very definite *physical sensations.* Whenever your body moves, you can feel it. Directing your attention to the natural, rhythmic movements of your breath and the accompanying physical sensations is very soothing. It has a profound tranquilizing effect on your mind and body.

Just notice: Can you feel any movement in your chest or in your belly as you slowly inhale and exhale? How about your back? Does any part of your back move as you breathe?

- You may feel very distinct physical sensations at this time, or you may feel nothing in particular. It really doesn't matter. Just be as you are, and see what you feel.

Step 5. *Your ribs expand as you breathe.* Now turn your attention to the ribs on your left side. Notice how those ribs move as you breathe. As you slowly inhale, your ribs swell and expand. As you exhale, your ribs relax.

If the expansion of your ribs isn't clear to you, you may place your left hand there to help you feel the ribs as they move. Can you feel anything there, even the slightest stirring, each time you inhale or exhale?

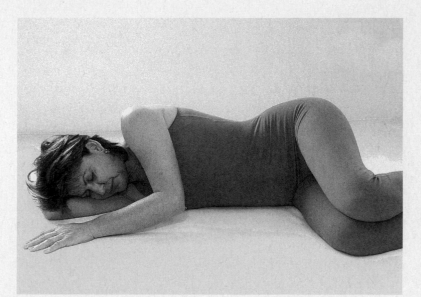

YOUR RIBS EXPAND AS YOU BREATHE. As you slowly inhale, your ribs swell and expand. As you exhale, your ribs relax.

Take your hand away from your ribs and rest. Can you feel that rhythmic movement of your ribs now, even without the help of your hand? You inhale, and your ribs rise toward the ceiling. They swell and expand. Then you exhale, and your ribs relax. They return to their resting state. This is one of the natural movements of the breath.

Step 6. *Your shoulder moves as you breathe.* Continue on your right side, as before. Now direct your attention to your left *shoulder*. As you slowly inhale, see if you can detect any movement, no matter how small or subtle, of your left shoulder. Each time you inhale, your shoulder moves a little bit in a certain direction. Each time you exhale, your shoulder returns to its starting position. As before, your breath produces the movement, not you.

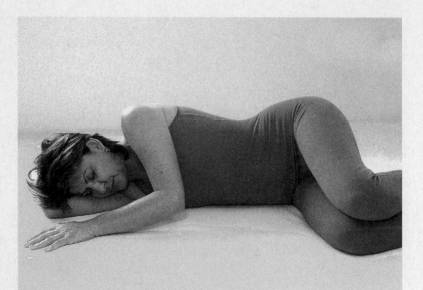

YOUR SHOULDER MOVES AS YOU BREATHE. As you slowly inhale, see if you can detect any movement of your shoulder, no matter how small or subtle.

- Why does your shoulder move like that? It makes perfect sense, really. Anytime a thing expands, it needs room to expand into. If there isn't room available, something else has to move aside in order to "make room."

- When you breathe in, your lungs fill with air, and as a result your ribs expand. As your ribs expand, they very gently *ease* the shoulder a little bit upward, toward your head. Your shoulder is "making room" for the expansion of your ribs.
- "Making room" is one of the fundamental principles of the Sounder Sleep System. Your body needs room. Room to breathe. Room to move. Room to live. When your body is cramped, crowded, and contracted, either internally or externally, you can't enjoy full aliveness. When your body is *spacious*, life is sweeter and easier, and your best self emerges without any effort.
- This is a special kind of mindful movement exercise. People nowadays don't often pay such close attention to the movements of their own breath. That's unfortunate, because your body really needs *close attention* from you. Your body needs your *attention and care*. When you pay *close attention* to your body, you are meeting one of its most fundamental needs. You are loving and caring for yourself. Loving and caring for your own body creates a sense of ease and well-being. This is the essence of self-nurturing. It doesn't take any scientific research to confirm this. You can experience it and know it directly with your own senses. That's very scientific!

So again, breathe easily and notice what happens. You inhale, the ribs on your left side expand, and your left shoulder moves a little bit to "make room" for the expansion of your ribs. You slowly exhale, your ribs relax, and your shoulder moves back the way it came. That is one of the natural, rhythmic movements of your living, breathing body. Isn't it wonderful?

The movement may be small and barely perceptible, or it may

be quite expansive and easy to feel. Whether the movement is big or small, it really doesn't matter as long as you direct your attention to each breath, each movement, each moment. Do that, and you'll master the Mini-Moves in no time at all.

Step 7. *Rest and reflect.* Rest a moment, and see how you feel now. Notice how your body rests against the bed or mat now. Notice how your head lies on the pillow. Is there any change, even a subtle one, in your mood, or in the quality of your thoughts?

- In a healthy, vital person, mind and body exist as a unified whole sharing a common rhythm. Sometimes, as a result of trauma, illness, prolonged stress, or ill-coordinated action, our minds and bodies get out of sync. As a result our actions assume an awkward quality, our thoughts become fragmented and unclear, and we feel irritable, uneasy, out of sorts. When that happens, our faculty for restful, restorative sleep is often one of the first things to suffer.
- This Mini-Move can help you to re-synchronize the rhythms of your mind and body, thereby restoring your mind and body to wholeness. When your mind and body are in sync, sleep is easy and complete.

Step 8. *Your hip moves as you breathe.* Now, just as we were exploring the movement of your left shoulder, let's explore also the movement of your left hip. For simplicity's sake, we'll define the *hip* as the highest point on the left side of your body when you're lying on your right side. So, slowly inhale, taking all the time you need for each breath. Your ribs expand, and the left side of your trunk rises a little bit toward the heavens. As your ribs expand like that, is there any movement, no matter how modest, of your left hip?

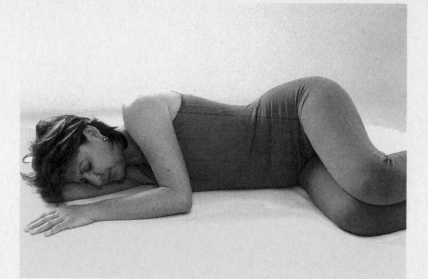

YOUR HIP MOVES AS YOU BREATHE. As you slowly inhale, see if you can detect any movement of your hip, no matter how small or subtle.

It may be that as you inhale like that, nice and easy, your ribs need some room to expand, and as a result, they ease the hip a little bit out of the way, to make room for a full inspiration. Stay with it for several breath cycles, and see what you discover. Make no effort to breathe deeply, or any special way. Make no intentional movement of your hip. If there is to be any movement, it will be a result of your breath only, and not any intentional action on your part.

Step 9. *The side of your body lengthens as you breathe.* Continue to rest quietly, and attend to your breathing and the movement of your ribs, your shoulder, and your hip.

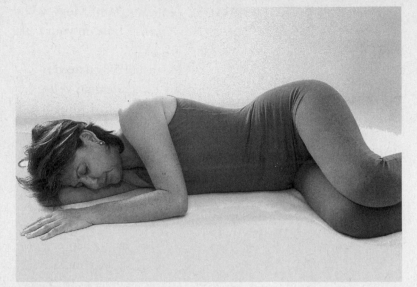

THE SIDE OF YOUR BODY LENGTHENS AS YOU BREATHE. Each time you inhale, the whole side of your body grows longer. Each time you exhale, you deeply relax.

See if you can feel the movement of your ribs, shoulder, and hip all at once: As you inhale, your ribs expand; they rise up toward the heavens, and as they do so, they ease the shoulder a little bit up, toward your head, and they ease the hip a little bit down, toward your feet. The hip and the shoulder move apart to "make room" for the expansion of your ribs as you breathe. You don't have to do anything—the movement happens all by itself.

When that happens, the whole left side of your torso grows longer, doesn't it? You breathe in, and your body grows longer, you breathe out, and you relax.

Step 10. *Rest and reflect.* Please lie on your back and rest quietly for a while. See if you can feel the difference between the left side of your body and the right. Does one side feel a little freer and more spacious?

When you are ready, you can repeat this Mini-Move while lying on your left side. When you have finished, lie on your back again and compare the two sides again.

Application. Practice this Mini-Move whenever you need to rest or recuperate from the stress of life. Since there are no voluntary movements involved, it's *extremely* restful. Done first thing in the morning, it will help you to establish a slow, easy rhythm for work or play. In the afternoon, it's the perfect prelude to a dreamy, restorative nap.

At bedtime, it will help you shift your attention away from the outer world of things and people, and into the welcoming depths of your own innermost self. You may combine this Calming Mini-Move with any of the Lulling Mini-Moves in chapter 5. Do ten minutes of Making Room. Then, still lying on your side, try Tongue in Cheek or the Ziggurat. Then rest a while. In the morning, you may not even recall the sequence of movements that carried you so sweetly to the shores of sleep.

Calming Mini-Move #3: Things Are Looking Up!

As a child I didn't like needles. When I needed to have a tooth filled I told my dentist that I wanted to do it without anesthesia—no needle! He said okay, he'd give it a try, and he started drilling, very slowly. That's when this Mini-Move was born. As the drill got close to the nerve, I gently rolled my eyes up. The drilling did hurt, but I found that I could relax and "not mind" quite so much. This simple expedient allowed me to endure the pain. I suppose my eyelids were open, because the dentist saw the whites of my eyes and stopped drilling. He thought I had fainted, so he was getting ready to wave some ammonia under my nose. It took us a little while to come to an understanding.

I have returned to this Mini-Move often over the years, and it has never failed to comfort me and lift my spirits. I have refined it considerably since that first discovery in the dentist's chair. Now I invite you to try it. You, too, can peacefully coexist with pain, stress, tension, anxiety—even depression. It will calm your mind and quell some of that mental chatter that robs you of your inner peace. For best results, practice a few minutes every day, morning and night. After a few weeks of that you will say, with all your heart, "Things are looking up!"

Step 1. *Get comfortable.* Sit in a chair or lie quietly on your back, and softly close your eyes. Notice the feeling in your lips, your cheeks, your forehead. Does your face feel at ease, or is it tense and contracted?

- Notice your eyes. Do your eyelids flutter slightly, even though your eyes are closed? Do your eyes move about? How about your forehead and your brow? Is your brow at rest, or is there some tension, some remnant of action or expression there? You needn't change anything. Just see what is.
- How about your eyes? Are your eyes fully at rest, or do they move about behind your closed lids? Where do your eyes come to rest when you're not actively looking at something? Do your eyes tend to go upward, or downward, or to one side or the other?

Step 2. *Raise your eyebrow with ease.* Softly close your eyes. Then slowly and gently raise and lower your *right* eyebrow several times. Is the movement smooth and continuous, or is it somewhat jerky or awkward?

- Your left eyebrow may want to move along with your right eyebrow. If so, don't stop it. Allow it to move, or not— whichever is easiest for you.

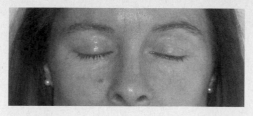

RAISE YOUR EYEBROW WITH EASE. Slowly and gently raise and lower one eyebrow several times. If your other eyebrow moves, too, that's fine.

- If you feel any discomfort or unease while moving your eyebrow like that, please do much smaller, easier movements. Reduce the range of your movements by half, and then by half again, until you feel that you can do small, easy movements with a sense of ease, lightness, and pleasure. When your movements are easy, light, and pleasurable, you are most receptive to discovering new options for action.

Stop and rest for a few moments.

This time, synchronize the movements of your eyebrow with your breath: Slowly inhale, and raise your right eyebrow. Slowly exhale, and allow your eyebrow to relax. Repeat several times. Does synchronizing the movement with your breath make it smoother and more continuous, or not?

When you move like that, do you tend to incline your head a little bit forward or back? See what you discover. Slowly inhale, raise your right eyebrow, and see which way your head tends to move.

Stop, rest, and feel the effect. Has there been any change in feeling of your forehead, your eyes, your lips, your cheeks? Does your right eyebrow feel different from its partner? Does the right side of your face feel different from the left?

Step 3. *Raise your eyelid with ease.* Slowly and gently raise and lower your right eyelid several times. You raise your eyelid, and your eye opens a little. You relax your eyelids, and your eyes softly close.

RAISE YOUR EYELID WITH EASE. Slowly and gently raise and lower one eyelid several times.

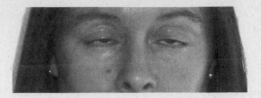

- When you raise your right eyelid, your left eyelid may want to move, too. Do not be concerned. Just let it move, or not— whichever is easier for you.

Attend to the quality of the movement of your eyelid. Is the movement smooth, easy, and gradual, or is it a bit awkward and jerky? Does your eyelid flutter as it moves? Don't try to do it differently—just observe what is.

Pause a moment and feel the effect.

This time, synchronize the movements of your eyelid with your breath. Slowly inhale, and raise your right eyelid; your eye softly opens. Slowly exhale, and allow your eyelid to relax; your eye softly closes.

Repeat several times. Does synchronizing the movement with your breath make it smoother and more continuous?

Stop, rest, and feel.

Step 4. *Raise your eyes with ease.* Softly close your eyes. With your eyes closed, slowly, gently allow your right eyeball to float upward, as if you were looking up, just above the horizon. Then, as you exhale, relax your eye. Continue. Do the movement several times more, pausing to rest and feel after each repetition.

RAISE YOUR EYES WITH EASE. With your eyes closed, slowly, gently allow one eyeball to float upward, as if you were looking up, just above the horizon. Then, as you exhale, relax your eye.

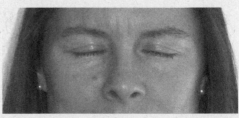

- Of course, when you move your right eye the left eye will move, too. For now, just keep your attention on your right eye, and let your left eye move of its own accord. No special effort is required.
- Your eyelids remain closed, but your eyeball rolls upward as if you were looking up. Do small movements, with a minimum of effort. Just allow your eyes to float upward.
- If you feel any discomfort when you raise your eyes like that, please do the movement in your imagination only. When you imagine your eye moving, it moves ever so slightly in the direction that you imagine. For our purposes, those tiny, effortless, imaginary eye movements are just as effective as actual ones.

Stop, rest, and feel the result of what you have done.

Continue moving your right eye as before, but this time, synchronize the movement of the eye with your breath. Slowly inhale, raise your right eye up. Slowly exhale, and relax your eye. Repeat several times.

When you move like that, do you tend to incline your head a little bit in a certain direction? See what you discover. Slowly inhale, allow the right eye to float upward, and see which way your head tends to move. Backward, or forward?

Stop, rest quietly, and feel the effect of what you have done. Notice how your eyes, eyelids, and eyebrows feel now.

Step 5. *Put it all together.* Now, if you're still awake, we'll combine the movements of the eyebrow, eyelid, and eye into a single, effortless gesture. We'll take it in two stages.

Stage 1: Slowly raise your right eyebrow. Notice that as your eyebrow rises higher, it gently tugs at your right eyelid, encouraging it to rise, too. It's as if the rising eyebrow were dragging the lid open ever so slightly. Then, relax your eyebrow, and allow your eyelid to close. Repeat several times.

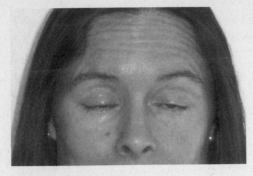

PUT IT ALL TOGETHER. Combine the movements of the eyebrow, eyelid, and eye into a single, effortless gesture.

Continue, synchronizing the movement with your breath. Slowly inhale, raise your right eyebrow, then your right eyelid. Slowly exhale, relax the brow, and relax the eyelid. Repeat several times.

- Pause for a few moments and feel the result of what you've done. Breathe easy, and think of nothing in particular.

Stage 2: Slowly inhale, and as you do so, gently raise your right eyebrow, followed by your right eyelid. As you do that, do you notice your right eye moving a little bit in a certain direction?

That's right: Just as the rising eyebrow invites the eyelid to rise along with it, the raising of both the eyebrow and the eyelid invites the eye itself to float upward. See if you can move the three parts in a sequential manner: first the eyebrow, next the eyelid, then the eye.

Do several movements like that. Slowly inhale, raise the right eyebrow, raise the eyelid, raise the eye. Slowly exhale, then relax the brow, relax the lid, and relax the eye. Repeat several times.

Stop, rest, and feel the result of what you have done.

Do you feel differently than before? At this point, many people tell me that their eyelids feel like heavy blankets covering their eyes. Notice how still your eyes have become. Do you feel like cracking a yawn? Be my guest!

Step 6. *Continue as before.* Slowly inhale, and as you do, allow your eyes to float upward. Slowly exhale, and as you do, let your eyes return to their natural resting position. Pause and feel the effect. Repeat several times, pausing after each movement. Then stop, rest, and feel.

- Notice how quiet your mind has become. When *feeling* takes the place of *thinking,* the mind becomes very tranquil. Linger there as long as you like, savoring that feeling of inner peace and tranquility.

Step 7. *To conclude.* Now, as you did at the beginning: Very, very slowly raise and lower your eyelids several times. How does it feel to raise and lower your eyelids now? Is the movement a little smoother, a little easier, a little softer? The quality of the movement of your eyelids is a reliable barometer of your personal stress quotient. When you can move your eyelids smoothly, easily, softly, you can assume that your body is at ease and your mind is at peace.

Application. Your body and mind have their own built-in system for sustaining pleasure and moderating pain. This Mini-Move allows you to mobilize that self-healing system whenever you feel the need. You can attain a state of serenity anytime, anywhere. It brings you pleasure and peace. Isn't it nice to know that your most powerful resources for self-healing are right there within yourself?

Calming Mini-Move #4: Main Squeeze

This Mini-Move and the one that follows both employ a special way of joining your hands that I light-heartedly call the Secret Handshake. Of course, there's nothing secret about it—I have been teaching it to people all over the United States and in Europe for years. Karen Bonime, a seasoned elementary school teacher, attended my four-part introductory course in Albuquerque. At the end of the course, she confessed that she had taught this Mini-Move to her entire fourth-grade class. Of course, I was delighted.

"We all love the Secret Handshake," reports Ms. Bonime. "We use it to help the children calm down when they're coming back into the room after an assembly or a play period, and to relieve pre-testing jitters. And when the children notice me getting flustered or upset, someone is bound to remind me: 'Ms. Bonime! Ms. Bonime! You'd better do the Secret Handshake!'"

I myself used to practice the Secret Handshake, and especially this variation of it called the Main Squeeze, during rush hour on the New York City subway. I found that I could shut out all the noise and crowding and arrive at a place of profound stillness in the midst of all that chaos. I used to have some of my most peaceful times right there, on the A train. I have taught the Main Squeeze to people from every walk of life—lawyers and cops, seniors and teenagers, artists and executives—all with remarkable results. I hope you'll find a place in your daily routine for this wonderful self-healing practice. May it serve you well!

PART ONE: THE SECRET HANDSHAKE

Step 1. *Get ready.* Find a comfortable chair to sit on. It's a good idea to remove your shoes if you can. You may find it helpful to place a pillow or a folded blanket in your lap for this Mini-Move.

Sit upright on the front half of the seat, if that is comfortable for you. If it's not, sit any way that you can. If your legs are crossed, uncross them and place the soles of your feet flat on the floor. If you need a pillow to support your lower back, go and get it. Make yourself as comfortable as you can.

Step 2. *Check in.* Take a few moments to check in with yourself. What do you notice while you're sitting like that? You may want to close your eyes to make it easier to feel.

- Feel the way the soles of your feet make contact with the floor. The right sole; the left sole.
- Feel the way your bottom makes contact with the chair. Do you sit balanced, or does more of your weight rest on one side?
- How about your shoulders? Are they at ease or not? Are your cheeks, lips, eyes in repose? You needn't change anything at this time. Just notice how it is.
- Notice the feeling in your hands. Do your hands feel warm or cool?

Step 3. *Extend your hands.* Extend your hands in front of you with the palms facing down.

Step 4. *Grasp your thumb.* Move your hands together and grasp one of your thumbs from above, as if you were holding the handlebar of a bicycle. Both palms should still be facing down.

- Hold whichever thumb you prefer. Most people have a preference for holding one thumb or the other. Hold the thumb that feels most comfortable and natural for you. Which thumb is that, the right or the left? That will be the one you hold throughout this Mini-Move.

SECRET HANDSHAKE 1.
Place your hands in front of
you with the palms facing
down.

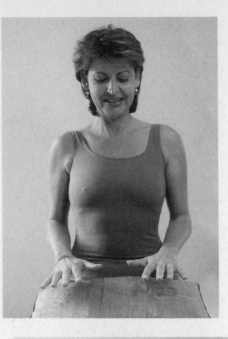

SECRET HANDSHAKE 2.
Move your hands together and
grasp one of your thumbs.

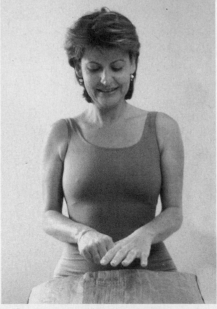

Step 5. *Extend your index finger.* Which hand do you use to grasp your thumb? With that same hand, extend the index finger, as if to point at something in front of you.

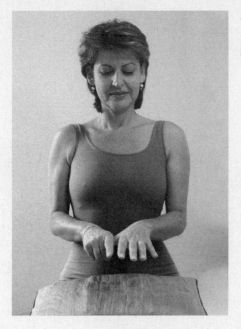

SECRET HANDSHAKE 3.
Extend the index finger of the grasping hand.

Step 6. *Grasp your index finger.* Bring the four fingers of the other hand over the extended index finger, and grasp it. You are now grasping your thumb with one hand, and your index finger with the other hand.

Step 7. *Lower your hands.* Keeping your hands joined like that, allow them to rest in your lap so that your arms, wrists, and hands are comfortably supported. Relax your hands as much as possible. There's no need to grip or squeeze.

SECRET HANDSHAKE 4.
Grasp the extended index
finger with the fingers of the
other hand.

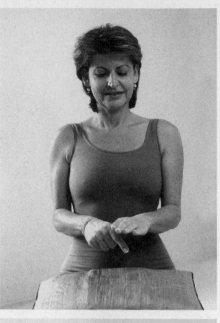

SECRET HANDSHAKE 5.
Keeping your hands joined as
above, allow them to rest in
your lap. Relax your hands.
There's no need to grip or
squeeze.

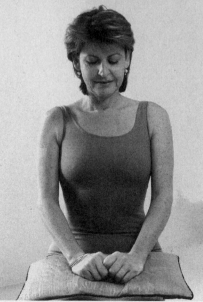

- Take a few moments to see how that feels. Some people find that simply holding their hands in this position is very comforting. They say it produces a feeling of ease and tranquility.

Step 8. *Feel the sensation.* Sit quietly and attend to the sensation you feel in your hands, in your index finger, and in your thumb. Closing your eyes makes it easier to feel.

Breathe naturally. Take all the time you need for each breath. You may discover a wide variety of sensations there, in your hands. You may feel warmth, a gentle pulsation, or a pleasant tingling or radiating sensation. You are a living, breathing, ever-moving being.

PART TWO: SQUEEZING YOUR THUMB

Step 9. *Squeeze and relax.* Now slowly inhale and, as you do so, gently, gradually squeeze your thumb. Then slowly exhale and gradually relax your grip on the thumb.

- Make the squeezing movement gentle and gradual. As long as you can feel the squeeze, that's enough.

Repeat the movement several times. Inhale, squeeze the thumb; exhale, and relax your grip.

Step 10. *Notice the feeling.* Keeping your hands joined like that, stop, rest, and feel. Let your breathing be nice and easy. Relax your hands as much as possible. Notice the feeling there.

- You may find that the pleasant sensation of warmth, pulsation, or radiating in your fingers and hands is more pronounced now than before. If so, that's an indication that you are becoming deeply relaxed.

- You may also feel that pleasant sensation migrating to your wrists, your arms, your shoulders. Take a moment to acknowledge any pleasurable bodily sensations that you may feel. By inviting those pleasurable sensations, by welcoming them and savoring them, you are initiating the self-healing process. Diffuse, sustained, pleasurable bodily sensations are your key to self-healing and inner peace.

PART THREE: SQUEEZING YOUR INDEX FINGER

Step 11. *Squeeze and relax.* This time, slowly inhale and as you do, gently, gradually squeeze your index finger. Then exhale and as you do, gradually relax your grip on the finger. Repeat the movement several times. Inhale, squeeze the index finger; exhale, and relax.

Step 12. *Breathe normally. Stop, rest, and feel.* Notice the result of the movements you have done. Let your breathing return to normal.

PART FOUR: ALTERNATELY SQUEEZING THE THUMB AND THE INDEX FINGER

Step 13. *Alternate squeezes.* This time, you will squeeze the thumb and index finger on alternate breaths. Slowly inhale, and as you do so, gradually squeeze your thumb. Exhale, and gradually relax your grip. Then slowly inhale, and squeeze your index finger. Exhale, and relax your grip.

Repeat the movement several times, alternating between the thumb and the index finger. Inhale, squeeze the thumb; exhale, and relax. Inhale, squeeze the finger; exhale, and relax.

Step 14. *Stop, rest, and feel.* Notice the result of what you have done. Let your hands be completely at ease. Do your hands feel warm or cool now?

- You will find that after just a few rounds of this gentle movement alternating with periods of quiet rest, your mind becomes very calm and still.
- If at any time you feel your mind racing, or you are distracted by troubling thoughts, simply do the movement a few more times. You will regain your focus very quickly.

PART FIVE: RAISING YOUR EYES

Step 15. *Continue as before.* This time, each time you inhale and squeeze, allow your eyes to float upward. Your eyelids remain closed, but you raise your eyes as if you were looking up. Then exhale, relax your eyes, and relax your grip.

- Please make the movement of your eyes very easy and light. If moving your eyes that way causes any discomfort, move the eyes in your imagination only. For our purposes imaginary eye movements will be just as effective as real ones.

Repeat the movement several times. Inhale, squeeze your thumb, raise your eyes up. Exhale, relax your eyes, relax your grasp on the thumb. Inhale, squeeze your index finger, raise your eyes up. Exhale, relax your eyes, and relax your grip on the finger.

Step 16. *Stop, rest, and feel.* Notice the result of what you have done. Let your hands be very soft and relaxed.

- Notice the pleasurable sensations in your fingers, hands, wrists, and arms now. Do your hands feel warmer than before? Notice the feeling in your chest, your belly, your back. See if you can identify pleasurable sensations anywhere in your body. It's nice to be alive, isn't it?
- Notice your breathing now. Does it seem different in some way? Easy, natural breathing is soft, quiet, and effortless.

To conclude your practice, very gradually, as if by one molecule at a time, separate your hands and place them comfortably in your lap. Then very slowly open your eyes. There you are!

Application. To get yourself started on the path to sounder sleep, practice this Calming Mini-Move for at least ten minutes, three times a day. The effect is cumulative: The more you practice, the better the results. Your thoughts will become more positive, your creativity will flourish, and you will see a more beautiful person in the mirror!

Note: If you find that you become drowsy while practicing the Main Squeeze, or any other Relaxing Mini-Move during the day, you may do this Mini-Move with your eyes open. You'll remain lucidly alert and at the same time deeply relaxed.

Calming Mini-Move #5: A Twist of the Wrists (Movement Meditation for Daytime Relaxation)

This Calming Mini-Move employs the same Secret Handshake that we used in the previous Mini-Move. Please review that if necessary before you begin.

Step 1. *Get comfortable.* Find a comfortable chair to sit on. You may remove your shoes if you like. For this mini-move you may find it helpful to place a small pillow in your lap.

Sit upright on the front half of the seat, if that is comfortable for you. If it's not, sit any way that you can. If you need a pillow to support your back, you may use one. Uncross your legs and place the soles of your feet flat on the floor. Make yourself as comfortable as possible.

Step 2. *Observe yourself in repose.* Take a few moments to observe yourself. What do you notice while you're sitting like that? You may want to close your eyes to make it easier to feel.

- Feel the way the soles of your feet make contact with the floor. The right sole; the left sole. Feel the way your bottom makes contact with the chair. Do you sit balanced, or does more of your weight rest on one side?
- How about your shoulders? Are they at ease or not? Are your cheeks, lips, eyes in repose? You needn't change anything. Just notice how it is.
- Notice the feeling of your hands. Do your hands feel warm or cool?

Step 3. *Join your hands.* Join your hands in the Secret Handshake, as in the Main Squeeze, and lower your hands to your lap. Sit quietly and attend to the sensation you feel in your index finger and thumb. You may want to close your eyes to make it easier to feel. You may discover a wide variety of sensations such as warmth, a pulsation, or a pleasant tingling or radiating sensation there in your hands.

You may feel that pleasant sensation migrating to your wrists, your arms, your shoulders. Take a moment to acknowledge any pleasurable bodily sensations that you may feel. Pleasurable sensations are your key to self-healing and inner peace.

- As you sit like that, allow your breathing to be easy, light, and natural. Make no special effort to inhale or exhale. Effort is an obstacle to natural breathing.
- After each exhalation is complete, you may notice a slight pause before the next inhalation begins. In that brief moment when your breath is "empty," let your mind be very still. The next breath will come to you sweetly, in its own good time. You don't have to do a thing. Take your time with this. The whole world may be hurried, worried, and harried. You needn't be.

THE SECRET HAND-SHAKE. Begin by joining your hands in the Secret Handshake as illustrated in the preceding Mini-Move.

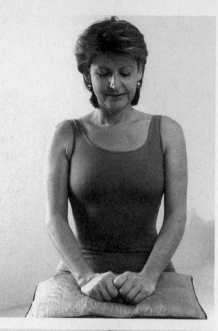

A TWIST OF THE WRISTS. Slowly inhale and, as you do so, gently, gradually bend your wrists a little bit back, so your knuckles rise upward and the backs of your hands incline very slightly toward you.

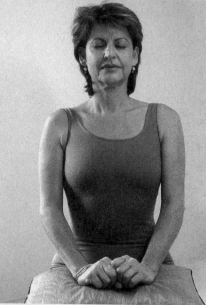

Step 4. *A twist of the wrists.* This time, slowly inhale and, as you do so, gently, gradually bend your wrists a little bit back, so your knuckles rise upward and the backs of your hands incline very slightly toward you. Then slowly exhale and gradually relax your wrists, allowing your hands to come to rest in your lap as before.

Your wrists and forearms remain supported in your lap all the while. As you inhale, your wrists bend back very slightly, and your knuckles rise up a little bit. Then, as you exhale, your wrists relax and your hands come to rest in your lap.

- Make your movements light and easy. As long as you can feel a little movement in your wrists, that's enough. For our purposes, light, easy, minimal movements are far more effective than big, powerful ones.

Repeat the movement several times. Inhale, bend the wrists; exhale, and relax the wrists. Continue.

- Synchronize your movements with your breathing. That means however long it takes you to slowly inhale, that's how long it takes you to gradually bend your wrists a little bit. However long it takes you to slowly exhale, that's how long it takes you to gradually relax your wrists and let your hands come to rest in your lap.

Step 5. *Stop, rest, and feel.* Let your breathing be easy and soft. Keeping your fingers joined as before, relax your hands as much as possible. Notice the feeling there.

- You may find that the sensation of warmth, pulsation, or radiating in your fingers and hands is more pronounced now than before. If so, that's an indication that you are becoming deeply relaxed.

You have now learned the basic movements of a Twist of the Wrists. Practice regularly, and you will enjoy all the benefits. Later, you may wish to try the following variation. The eye movements will be easier for you if you have practiced Things Are Looking Up! earlier in this chapter.

Step 6. *Raise your eyes.* This time, slowly inhale and bend your wrists, and simultaneously allow your eyes to float upward. Your eyelids remain closed, but you allow your eyes to move upward, as if you were looking up. Then exhale, relax your eyes, and relax your wrists.

- Please do make the movement of your eyes very easy and light. If moving your eyes this way causes any discomfort at all, move your eyes in imagination only. For our purposes imaginary eye movements are just as effective as real ones.

Continue. Inhale, bend your wrists, let your eyes float upward. Exhale, relax your eyes, and relax your wrists.

Step 7. *Stop, rest, and feel.* Notice the result of the movements you have done.

- Notice the pleasant sensation in your fingers, hands, and wrists now. If you pay close attention, you may find that the feeling spreads up your arms, deep into the core of your body. You may feel it somewhere in your chest, your belly, your hips, your back, or anywhere in your body. Diffuse, sustained, pleasurable body sensations are the key to self-healing and inner peace. They are your ever-present reminder of the joy of being alive.
- After just a few rounds of this gentle movement alternating with periods of quiet rest, your mind becomes very calm and still. If at any time you feel your mind racing, or if you be-

come distracted by troubling thoughts, simply do the movement a few times more. You will regain your focus very quickly.

Application. To get yourself started on the path to sounder sleep, practice this Calming Mini-Move for at least ten minutes, three times a day. The best times to practice are upon rising, before lunch, in the late afternoon, just before bed, or any time you could use a respite from the stress of life. The effect is cumulative: The more you practice, the better the results. Your thoughts will become more positive, your creativity will flourish, and you will see a more beautiful person in the mirror!

Note: If you find that you become drowsy while practicing during the day, you may do this Mini-Move with your eyes open. You'll remain lucidly alert and at the same time deeply relaxed.

Calming Mini-Move #6: Touching Your Heart

Terry was the nervous type. At the time of our first meeting, my office was being painted, so I had rented a small treatment room at TRS, a suite of commercial offices on the East Side. Our appointment was my first of the day, at 9:00 a.m. I arrived at 8:50 to find Terry in an altercation with the receptionist. It seems he had presented himself for a nine o'clock appointment with me and had been informed that that was impossible because no room was booked in my name until 9:30. He had become very agitated. He was on a tight schedule, and a half-hour delay was not acceptable to him. And he had let everyone around him know it! His face was bright red, his breath was quick and shallow, and he compulsively clenched and unclenched his right hand—all physiological signs of stress and anxiety.

It took me only a minute to sort things out with the TRS staff. They had made a mistake and were only too happy to give us a much larger room usually reserved for meetings and workshops.

There was no problem. In fact, we were far more comfortable than we would have been without the mistake. Our session began at 9:01.

I asked Terry if he was satisfied with the way he had handled the situation. He admitted that it wasn't his best moment. It seemed that he was in the habit of "going off," as he termed it. The smallest little glitch would send him into a tizzy—a cab that didn't stop for him, a meeting that went overtime, a delivery man who brought the wrong take-out order—and he'd become anxious and combative. He worked in the computer department of a large law firm, and he had been cited for his outbursts there.

We spent the rest of our session reenacting several situations that had triggered Terry in the past, starting with the most recent example that morning. In each case, I asked Terry to try to catch himself at the tipping point, where he was just on the verge of going off. At that moment, I asked him to bring his hand to his heart and for sixty seconds to just feel the warmth there. Each time we got to the tipping point, I could see Terry's ears start to redden and his breath start to accelerate. Then, at first with my prompting, and later on his own, he'd bring his hand to his heart and the process would come to a halt. Within a minute, he was calm and could address the situation in a more dispassionate way.

Terry understood immediately that this was a way to interrupt his habitual stress response. He was quite pleased with the results of our experiments. Later that day, he was tested under battlefield conditions. His supervisor criticized some code he had written and he caught himself at the moment he was starting to go off.

"Right there in front of my supervisor, I put my hand on my heart," Terry reported, "and I felt calm." Then he chuckled. "You know what? It turned out I didn't even write that code. It was written by a guy who left the company months ago!" Terry became very adept at touching his heart in a variety of situations. His life became easier as a result. He began to enjoy it.

This Mini-Move is simple and delightful. Over time, it cultivates a feeling of inner peace, plus greater compassion for yourself and others. Let's hope it's contagious!

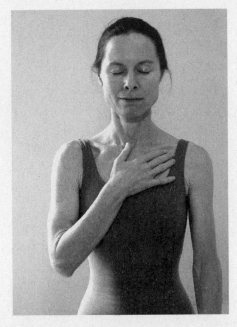

TOUCH YOUR HEART.
Place the center of the palm of one of your hands over the center of your chest.

Step 1. *Touch your heart.* Sit, stand, or lie down in any comfortable position. Place the center of the palm of one of your hands over the center of your chest. Find the warmest spot there.

Step 2. *Feel.* Feel the warmth of your hand as it meets the warmth of your heart. At first, it may take a moment or two for you to begin to feel it. Don't worry, it gets easier with practice. Don't hurry. Close your eyes if you like. Breathe easy.

- Which is warmer, your hand or your heart? Allow your heart to warm your hand and your hand to warm your heart.
- Each time you inhale, your chest rises and expands and your hand rises with your chest. Each time you exhale, your chest sinks and your hand sinks with it. Allow your hand to ride up and down with the gentle rising and falling of your chest.
- Continue touching your heart for several complete breath cycles.

Step 3. *Stop, rest, and feel.* Lower your hand and rest a moment. Don't hurry. Take all the time you need for each breath. Can you still feel the warmth there, in your chest?

Step 4. *Switch hands.* Try the same thing with the other hand. Simply touch your heart. Again, try to align the center of your palm with the warmest spot on your chest. Continue like that for as long as you like.

TOUCH YOUR HEART WITH BOTH HANDS. Place one hand over your heart, and the other hand on top of it. When the centers of both palms are aligned over the warmest spot on your chest, you will feel a core of warmth projecting from your hands, deep into the center of your chest.

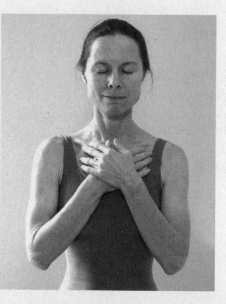

Step 5. *Touch your heart with both hands.* Place one hand over your heart and the other hand on top of it. When the centers of both palms are aligned over the warmest spot on your chest, you will feel a core of warmth projecting from your hands, deep into the center of your chest.

Make no effort. Breathe easy, and allow your hands to ride up and down with the gentle rising and falling of your breath.

Stop, rest, and feel.

Step 6. *Touch your heart with a smile.* Touch your heart with one or both hands, whichever you prefer. Allow your hands to ride up and down with the rising and falling of your breath. Now each time you slowly inhale, *think a smile*. Each time you exhale, relax. Continue for several breath cycles. It doesn't hurt, does it?

Step 7. *Circulate your smile.* Now, your lips aren't the only part of you that can smile. If there is some part of you that needs special care, you can send the image and the feeling of your smile there. It could be your stomach, your liver, your lungs, or your intestines. It could be your throat, your lower back, your head, or anywhere. You can circulate your smile around inside yourself, wherever you feel the need. Slowly inhale, and send your smile *there*. Slowly exhale, relax. You can concentrate on one area, or let your smile circulate all around your body.

Application. You can practice touching your heart anytime. You don't have to do all the steps every time. Sometimes just raising one hand to your heart for a brief moment is all it takes. That connects you to your inner self and to others, heart to heart. What more effective stress reducer could there be?

Chapter 5

★ ★ ★
★　　　★

Lull Yourself to Sleep

lull *vt* 1 : to cause to sleep or rest : SOOTHE 2 : to cause to relax
vigilance.
—WEBSTER'S NEW COLLEGIATE DICTIONARY

Sleep makes us forgetful of all things, of good and evil, when
once it has overshadowed our eyelids.
—THE ODYSSEY

Easy Steps Toward Natural, Restful Sleep

Congratulations! If you have read this far, and if you've practiced
some of the Mini-Moves in the two preceding chapters, you've
already made a good start on your quest for more natural, restful
sleep. You've begun to develop your innate ability to relax your
body and calm your mind, which, as we have seen, is your body's
built-in antidote to the deleterious effects of stress. You are now
amply prepared to learn the unique sleep-inducing Mini-Moves
that form the core of the Sounder Sleep System. Once you've
learned them, you will be able to do them right in your own bed
to lull yourself into a state of profound repose that's just right for a
delightful night of dozing and dreaming. Should you wake up
during the night, the Mini-Moves will help you to lull yourself

back to sleep quickly and easily. As a result, you'll get more of the natural, restful sleep you need, so you can start to enjoy life to the fullest. Yes, you can sleep through the night!

Just Joining Us?

If you *haven't* yet taken advantage of the preceding chapters and you're just plunging in now, welcome! You, too, will be able to follow the instructions and benefit from the sleep-induction techniques in this chapter. Please do be aware, however, that the Mini-Moves will have their greatest effect when used in concert with the physical and mental relaxation techniques presented in chapters 3 and 4. One of the key concepts of this book is that insomnia isn't just a bedtime problem, it's a problem that affects you twenty-four hours a day, whether you realize it or not. The physical and mental tension you experience during the course of the day doesn't just evaporate the moment you get into bed and close your eyes. Left unchecked, it overflows into your bedroom, keeping you wakeful at times you'd rather be fast asleep.

That's why it's so important to take some positive steps to reduce physical and mental tension during your waking hours. Reducing physical and mental tension during the day *sets the scene* for sounder, more restful sleep by making your life more peaceful and less stressful.

So if you haven't done so already, please consider backing up a step or two, and test-driving a few of the daytime Mini-Moves presented in each of the preceding chapters. At the very least, learn the soothing, exquisitely pleasurable Main Squeeze Mini-Move in chapter 4. Practice that for three to five minutes, three times a day, for a few days, and your life is bound to become sweeter and more livable. That will prepare you to enjoy all the benefits of the sleep-inducing Mini-Moves in this chapter.

The Path of No Effort

As you experiment with the Lulling Mini-Moves in this chapter, you will notice that I stress again and again the principle of *no effort*. This principle is articulated very clearly in the classic text of Taoist wisdom, the *Tao Te Ching:*

> Act without doing;
> work without effort.
> . . . Accomplish the great task
> by a series of small acts.
> —STEVEN MITCHELL, *trans.,*
> *Tao Te Ching, verse 63*

Though I first encountered this principle in my studies of the esoteric movement arts aikido, taiji, and qigong, and in my readings of Taoist texts like the *Tao Te Ching,* there is nothing esoteric about it! It is completely practical and immediately applicable to your personal quest for natural, restful sleep.

In fact, it's really just common sense, when you think about it: *Sleep is the antithesis of effort.* In order to sleep, we lie down, close our eyes, and *cease all activity.* While we sleep, we are incapable of voluntary action, incapable of making any effort. If that is so, how could we possibly expect to initiate the natural sleep process by making an effort? The path of sleep is the path of *no effort.* Sleep *begins* with the *cessation of all effort.*

While it is true that we must cease all effort in order to sleep, the converse is also true: *Making an effort to sleep can wake us up.* You see, the moment you decide that you are *not satisfied* with resting quietly, and that you *must* get to sleep immediately, you trigger a cascade of stress-related responses within yourself. Your heart beats a little faster, your muscles become tenser, your mind begins to mobilize itself in order to find a response to this challenge. When that happens, you already have departed from the path of no effort and are moving swiftly in the opposite direction, away from the Land of Nod.

In *Restful Sleep*, his invaluable book on the Ayurvedic approach to insomnia, Deepak Chopra writes eloquently of the futility of trying to force sleep. He advises the troubled sleeper to adopt an attitude of "not minding." By that he means simply resting quietly, "not minding whether you are awake or asleep." This is good advice, for two reasons. First, because just as the proverbial watched pot never boils, sleep rarely comes when you are watching for it. In fact, the very act of watching may keep you awake. Second, because any form of quiet rest, whether you sleep or not, is a balm to the body and the soul. A night of quiet rest is far more soothing and restorative than a night of anxious tossing and turning punctuated by periods of pacing the floor, late-night television, or Net surfing!

But relinquishing all effort is not all there is to it. We must also relinquish our *intention to control* the sleep process. "Our bodies are wild," writes Zen poet and environmentalist Gary Snyder in *The Practice of the Wild*. By that he means that the internal functions of our body are natural processes, like rain, wind, or continental drift. We may be "civilized" on the outside, but we're all wilderness inside. And as we all know, you can't control a wilderness—even with all the impressive technology in our hands, we still can't make rain fall or prevent tornadoes! Such things are governed by natural laws that are beyond our control.

Sleep is a feature of this internal wilderness of ours—and we can't control it, either. Like a wild beast, sleep comes and goes of its own accord. We cannot control it, but we can harmonize ourselves with its comings and goings and make ourselves ready for that mysterious moment when it does arrive. The alternative is to set our teeth and persist in trying to control that which cannot be controlled. Not only is that futile effort bound to fail, but it is also very likely to keep us awake long past our bedtime!

It's essential that we acknowledge these facts and act accordingly. That means taking the path of no effort: not trying to force ourselves to sleep, not interfering with the natural sleep.

But don't worry, you don't have to be a Taoist master to follow the path of *no effort*. Anyone can travel this pleasurable path to natural, restful sleep! That's because the principle of *no effort* is built right into each one of the Mini-Moves presented in this chapter. Simply follow the step-by-step instructions with their accompanying commentary, and you will spontaneously begin to travel the path of *no effort* toward sounder, more restful sleep. Without any special effort, your mind will become focused on "this breath, this movement, this moment." The past and present recede from your awareness, and you can just *be,* in the moment. Then, whatever your mind is holding on to, you can just let it go. You body relaxes, your mind gets calm and clear. Sleep will come to you sweetly, and you can welcome it with open arms.

The Pleasure Principle

In an enjoyable, popularly written book titled *Feeling Good Is Good for You,* Drs. Carl J. Charnetski and Francis X. Brennan document the healing powers of pleasure. The experience of pleasure, they explain, triggers the secretion of *endorphins*, the naturally occurring, opiate-like substances in your body that reduce inflammation and pain, relax your muscles, and bring you feelings of peace and well-being. Even better, this release of endorphins powers up your immune system, your body's innate self-healing mechanism. Consequently, if you're stressed out or facing illness or injury, the authors assert, the experience of pleasure can be a powerful ally in your healing process.

The most familiar example of the endorphin effect is the well-known "runner's high," which results when the stress of a good long run (or other vigorous workout) causes your body to secrete enough endorphins to cancel out the feelings of effort and strain associated with running and bring you to a state of physical pleasure and mental euphoria. That explains why, though we may feel stiff and unwilling at the beginning of a workout, we often experience a feeling of physical ease and mental well-being before it's over. It also highlights an important point: The endorphin effect is a palpable, physical experience. We can tell when we're secreting endorphins *because we can feel it with our own senses*.

Charnetski and Brennan have their own ideas about how to evoke pleasure for self-healing, and their approach runs to physical exercises like running or tennis and such warm, fuzzy pursuits as being with loved ones, playing with pets, singing, giving or receiving massage, and watching funny movies—all wonderful things, all practical, direct means for achieving pleasure. But these things probably won't help you at that mysterious moment when you're lying in bed, waiting for sleep to come. At that moment, you're alone with yourself and you need stillness, peace, and quiet so you can drift off to sleep.

Does that mean that pleasure is out of the picture? Are we to be denied, in that vulnerable moment, the benefit of nature's greatest power to comfort, to nurture, and to heal? Certainly not! Let me tell you something that Charnetski and Brennan don't say, something they may not even be aware of: Once you know how to live it, *pleasure is a perpetual state of being*. The healing, soothing endorphins—and any other substances that science in the future may identify as the chemical basis of our native sense of pleasure and ease—are circulating in your body at all times, whether you're aware of it or not. As a result, those *pleasurable feelings in your body* can be felt and enjoyed not only when you're actively running, singing, laughing, or petting the dog, but also when you're just being *very, very still*. In fact, those pleasurable bodily sensations can be experienced most acutely, most immediately, and with greatest enjoyment, at moments of profound stillness and tranquility, when you cease doing anything, and you simply *are*. These delicious feelings result from the simple fact of being alive, as expressed in the wondrous rhythmic movements of your own body and your own breath. And this is especially true at the moment when you are ready to drift off to sleep.

How will you know this is true? Do you have to take my word for it? No! You can easily confirm it for yourself. You will feel those soothing, pleasurable sensations in your own body, with your own senses, each time you do the Mini-Moves. And as you do, you will find that sleep comes to you easily, without any effort of will. Sweet dreams!

Guidelines for Your Practice of the Lulling Mini-Moves

The Lulling Mini-Moves presented in this chapter are specially designed exercises that you can do right in your own bed for deep relaxation, quiet rest, and sleep. Used in conjunction with the Relaxing and Calming Mini-Moves presented in chapters 3 and 4, they bring you to a state of profound mental and physical repose that's just right for drifting, dozing, and dreaming.

The Mini-Moves have been thoughtfully designed so that simply following the step-by-step instructions for each Mini-Move will bring you all the benefits. Even so, there are a few practical points that bear mentioning. The following tips will help you derive the maximum benefit from your practice of the Mini-Moves.

To begin, practice during waking hours. When you first practice the Mini-Moves they will be unfamiliar to you. The process of turning the pages of the book and reading and following the step-by-step instructions will require some thought and effort on your part. Thought and effort aren't conducive to sleep. Therefore, it's best to learn each Mini-Move by practicing it during waking hours. Later, when you can do the Mini-Move fluently, without thought or effort, you'll be ready to practice at bedtime.

Here's another reason for practicing during waking hours. If you have difficulty sleeping, bedtime may be a complicated experience for you. You may tend to wonder whether sleep will come and to worry about the consequences if it doesn't. What's more, all your habitual physical and emotional responses to sleep, what I call "sleep baggage," come to the surface at that moment. So, please begin your practice of these Lulling Mini-Moves during waking hours, *when nothing is at stake.* That way, you won't be so likely to be distracted by all your sleep baggage.

Later, practice every night at bedtime. Once you've learned a Lulling Mini-Move and are ready to practice at bedtime, practice a little bit every night. The Lulling Mini-Moves have a cumulative effect. The more you practice, the greater the benefit.

With regular nightly practice, the Lulling Mini-Moves will become second nature to you. That way, you can do them without thinking. *And the less you have to think, the more you'll be able to feel.* Feel the blissful sensation of your own living, moving, breathing body. Feel that sweet fatigue that invites you to slide into a sleepy, dreamy, drowsy state. When thinking is replaced by feeling, your body relaxes and your mind becomes calm and clear. From there, it's just a hop, skip, and jump to Dreamland.

If you're one of the many people who fall asleep easily at bedtime, but wake up during the night and have difficulty getting back to sleep, consistent bedtime practice of the Lulling Mini-Moves will be particularly helpful for you. By doing a Mini-Move at bedtime and then falling asleep as you normally do, you are conditioning your mind and body to fall asleep whenever you do those particular movements. That way, when you awaken during the night, just do the same Mini-Move for a few minutes. Soon enough, you will lie warm in the gold of dawn.

Rest. Every Mini-Move consists of alternating active and passive phases: gentle, synchronized *movements* alternating with periods of *quiet rest.* Believe it or not, these rest periods are the most important part of the Mini-Moves!

The movements are a stimulus that triggers your body's natural faculty for rest, relaxation, and sleep. But it's during the *rest periods* that your body receives the stimulus, processes it, and responds by becoming deeply relaxed. Each time you cease action and rest, the gentle waves of your breath wash you a little closer to the shores of sleep, a little deeper into the sleepy, dreamy drowsy state. Therefore, when the instructions say to rest, please rest. That will allow the Mini-Moves to have their best effect.

Rest well. By that I mean, don't skimp on the rest periods. In general, your rest periods should be about as long as the periods of movement that precede them, *or longer.* There's a simple way to monitor this. Let's say you do a sequence of eight movements, each one lasting a complete breath cycle (a breath cycle consists of an inhalation, an exhalation, and any pauses in between). The movement period would then be a total of eight complete breath cycles in duration. In that case your rest period, too, ought to last about eight full breath cycles *or more.*

When you begin, you may want to actually count the movements and breath cycles to give you a feeling for the lulling, rhythmic quality of the Mini-Moves. Later, you can abandon the counting and simply *breathe, move,* and *feel.* With regular practice of the Mini-Moves, you will begin to observe this rhythmic alternation of action and repose naturally, without even thinking about it.

Rest longer. As you become more adept in your practice of the Mini-Moves, allow yourself longer and longer rest periods following each set of movements. At the beginning, your rest periods may last three, five, seven, or eight *breath cycles.* Later, they may last three, five, seven, or eight *minutes.*

If at any time your mind starts racing or you become physically restless, begin another round of synchronized movements and breathing. You will regain your composure very quickly that way, and you can resume your quiet rest. The longer you can maintain that quiet resting state between the movements, the more likely you will be to drift into that sleepy, dreamy, drowsy state that's just right for restful, restorative sleep.

Make your movements light and easy. In my nearly twenty years as a movement educator, I've observed again and again that people almost always use more force than necessary to perform any given action, often with unexpected results. We shake hands so vigorously that we cause each other to wince in pain. We whack the computer keys so hard we damage our hands and wrists. We close the faucet so tight the washers wear out before their time. We seem to think that by working harder, by using more force, we'll get better results. But it isn't so!

When you first practice the Mini-Moves, it is very likely that you will tend to do the movements more vigorously than need be. You see, your everyday actions such as walking, hammering a nail, sweeping a floor, using a computer, or driving a car do require a certain amount of force to get the job done, and your nervous system is calibrated to function more or less within that range of forces. But the Mini-Moves are quite different from those everyday actions. When you do the Mini-Moves, you don't have to interact with any object. You don't have to do anything. You simply *move* and *breathe.* That requires only minimal force.

When you can stop doing and simply move and breathe with minimal effort, something very special happens. You begin to feel more acutely than ever before. You feel yourself, your body, and your breath in a new way. When you can withdraw your attention from the cares and concerns of the outside world and become immersed in the awareness of "this breath, this movement, this moment," you will find yourself slipping into a blissful slumber without any effort. That is the central principle upon which the Sounder Sleep System is based.

However, this quality of being is very unfamiliar to most people in this society. As a result, unless you have already had some special training in the art of movement, you probably will do the Mini-Moves with more force than necessary, at least at first. *Don't worry—the Mini-Moves will have an effect anyway!* But for best results, and for your greatest pleasure and enjoyment, try to gradually make your movements even lighter, even easier, even *softer* than anything you can imagine. One way to achieve this is to decrease the amplitude of your movements by half, and then by half again. Then, at the moment you feel that you really are doing the movements with *unimaginable* lightness and ease, that heavy curtain of darkness will fall over your eyes, and all will be peace.

Don't fight sleep. If you should feel sleepy at any time while learning these Mini-Moves, do not be concerned. That simply means that you have already absorbed as much as you can for the moment, and you are ready to rest. Don't fight it!

The urge to sleep is a direct expression of one of your body's most fundamental needs. Fighting sleep sends a message to your body that *its needs don't matter*. But the truth is, *your bodily needs do matter,* a lot. They are of inestimable importance in your quest for sounder sleep and a more restful, balanced life.

The reason is this: Whenever your thoughts and actions are in

perfect accord with your real needs, even if it's just for a ~~m~~
your body begins to heal itself. That's the fundamental ~~p~~
on which this book is based. The Mini-Moves are physical actions
that are in perfect accord with your needs, especially your need for
natural restful sleep. Whenever you do the Mini-Moves, you are
initiating a self-healing process that enables you to recover from
insomnia and the stress of life.

So, whenever you feel that sleepy, dreamy, drowsy feeling coming on, please do stop and take a little rest. *That is your real need!*
Getting the rest you need, *when you need it,* should always be your
highest priority. Once you are completely rested, you can begin
afresh. Learning at your own pace will ensure your fullest enjoyment of this program and the greatest possible benefit to you.

Lulling Mini-Move #1: Breath Surfing 1

> When you are about to fall asleep
> and all external objects have faded from view,
> concentrate on the state between sleep and waking.
> There the Supreme Goddess will reveal herself.
> —VIJNANABHAIRAVA, *verse 75*

Each breath you take is like a gentle wave on the ocean. Breath
Surfing is the art of catching those waves and riding them to the
shores of sleep. Once you have reached that sleepy, dreamy,
drowsy state, simply rest quietly and enjoy the scenery. The inner
wisdom of your own mind and body will decide what happens
next.

Step 1. *Observe yourself at rest.* Lie on your back in bed, or on a
soft mat or carpet on the floor. You can use a pillow to support
your head and neck if you like. Do whatever you need to get
comfortable.

- How does it feel to lie still like that? Do you feel relaxed and at ease or do you feel restless?
- Are your eyes at rest, or do they move about? How do you breathe? Does your breathing feel easy and free, or not?

Step 2. *Home position.* Now please bend your right elbow and bring the four fingertips of your right hand to lightly touch your sternum. (Your sternum is the vertical breastbone in the center of your chest, where the ribs come together.) Let your right thumb come to rest somewhere on your chest, wherever it falls naturally.

Now do the same thing with your left hand. The tips of the four fingers of both hands rest on either side of the sternum. Your thumbs rest comfortably anywhere on your chest.

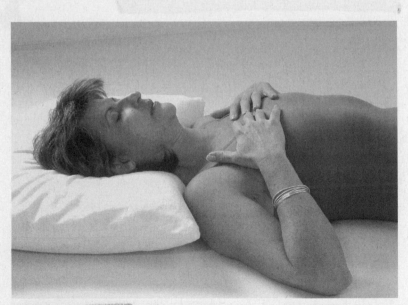

HOME POSITION. Breath surfing, home position. The tips of the four fingers of both hands rest on either side of your chest. Your thumbs rest wherever it's most comfortable for you.

- Allow your elbows to rest on the bed or floor in whatever way is most comfortable for you. Let your wrists, hands, and fingers be at ease. The tips of your fingers rest lightly on your sternum. Do not press. No force is required.

Step 3. *Observe the movements of your breath.* Slowly breathe in, and slowly breathe out. Each time you breathe in, your chest rises. Each time you breathe out, your chest sinks. Touching your sternum with your fingertips makes it easier to feel the movement of your body as you slowly inhale and slowly exhale.

- Don't try to accomplish anything at this point. Simply wait and see what you discover. Just breathe naturally, without trying to do anything special.

Take some time to become familiar with the natural rising and falling movement of your chest, no matter how modest that movement may be. Perhaps you don't feel anything special at this point. If so, that's perfectly okay. Just keep following along, and you will improve more than you can imagine.

- Continue resting quietly, and attend to any pleasurable sensation you may discover anywhere in your body.

Step 4. *Ride the breath with your thumbs.* Place the fingertips of both hands in the home position. Your thumbs rest comfortably anywhere on your chest.

Turn your attention to your thumbs, and the area of the chest directly underneath each thumb. Tune in to the movements of those little, localized areas of your chest under each thumb. Each time you slowly inhale, those parts of your chest rise and expand, and your thumbs rise and move with them. Each time you slowly exhale, your chest sinks, and your thumbs sink with your chest.

- Have you ever seen surfers sitting on their boards, waiting for a wave? Each passing swell lifts the surfers up and gently lowers them back down again. The movement is rhythmic and repetitive. The rising and falling of your chest is like that. This Mini-Move is very simple. You simply ride your chest up and down with your thumbs.

Make no effort to move your thumbs. The upward and downward movement of the thumbs is produced by the rhythmic rising and falling of the chest as you breathe.

NOW

Step 5. *Lift and lower your thumbs.* Slowly inhale. As your chest rises, slowly and gradually lift your thumbs away from your chest a little tiny bit.

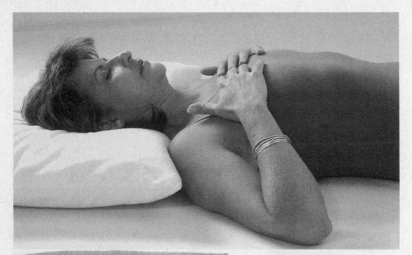

LIFT AND LOWER YOUR THUMBS. As your chest rises, slowly and gradually raise your thumbs away from your chest a little tiny bit. Slowly exhale, and relax your thumbs.

Then slowly exhale. Your chest falls. As you exhale, gradually relax the thumbs and let them come to rest on your chest.

- The lifting of the thumbs should be very soft, slow, and gradual. Raise the thumbs just enough that you can feel them break contact with your chest, no more. Use the minimum force necessary to lift the thumbs.

Repeat the movement several times. Slowly inhale, lift your thumbs. Slowly exhale, relax the thumbs, and let them come to rest.

- Synchronize the movements of your thumbs with your breath. That means, however long it takes you to breathe in, it takes that same amount of time to raise the thumbs. However long it takes you to breathe out, it takes that same amount of time to slowly lower the thumbs.
- See if you can you feel that moving your thumbs like that has a subtle influence on the movement of your chest as you breathe, either on the area of your chest directly beneath your thumbs or anywhere else.

Step 6. *Stop, rest, and feel.* Feel the result of what you have done. Let your breathing be light and easy. As you continue to rest quietly, notice how your thumbs rise and fall with the rising and falling of your breath *now*. You may find that the movement of your chest is a little freer, a little fuller, a little easier now. See what you discover.

Step 7. *Continue.* Repeat Steps 5 and 6 several times, as desired. Let the rest periods between the movements get longer and longer with each repetition.

The rest periods are the most important part of this Mini-Move. The movements are designed to stimulate your body-mind's innate ability to relax and sleep. It is during the rest periods that your body and mind receive the stimulus, process it, and respond by becoming deeply relaxed.

- You may dream, you may drift, you may linger in that sleepy, dreamy, drowsy state that's just right for rest, meditation, or sleep. Make no effort to fall asleep. Allow the inner wisdom of your own mind and body to decide what happens next.

Variation. Once you've relaxed yourself by doing the Breath Surfing technique described above, you may find it helpful to try the following variation. The subtle movements will help you achieve even greater tranquility and peace.

Step 8. *Lighten your thumbs.* Again, slowly inhale, and this time, lift your thumbs, but do it so delicately that they never break contact with your chest. As your chest rises, carrying the thumbs upward, you activate the muscles of your thumbs a tiny little bit, as if to make the thumbs a little lighter. You are lifting your thumbs without really lifting them. You're just *lightening* them.

Then, slowly exhale. As your chest sinks, relax your thumbs and allow them to be carried downward by your chest. Your chest and your thumbs remain perfectly synchronized and in full contact all the time. Repeat the movement several times, as desired.

Step 9. *Stop, rest, and feel.* Rest quietly for several complete breath cycles, and enjoy the stillness you've created within yourself. You may notice that the movement of your breath is a little softer, a little slower than when you began. Your body is relaxed, your mind is calm. Each new round of movements takes you a little deeper into a state of profound repose.

Step 10. *Continue.* Repeat Steps 4 through 9 as desired. Be sure to maintain the regular, alternating rhythm of the movements and breath: Do five, six, seven, or eight movements, then rest for an equal or greater number of breath cycles. You needn't count. The numbers are just a convenient guide.

Step 11. *Imagine the movements of the thumbs.* As you relax more and more deeply, you can Breath Surf as above, but simply imagine yourself lifting and lowering your thumbs with the breath. Make no voluntary movement of the thumbs, just imagine it.

For further practice: Once you've learned the basic technique, you can try all of these Breath Surfing variations with your index, middle, ring, or little fingers in place of the thumbs. Each finger gives a slightly different relaxing effect. You can also try Breath Surfing with your hands on the middle or lower breathing spaces. In time, you will find the way of Breath Surfing that suits you best. Sweet dreams!

Application. This simple exercise makes it easy to lull yourself into a state of deep tranquility. All the mental chatter, your mind's endless monologue, fades into the background. The past and the future recede from your awareness; the present moment is all there is. That timeless moment is your gateway to rest, meditation, introspection, dreams, or sleep, whichever is right for you in this moment.

Practice this Mini-Move every night when you get into bed, even if you tend to fall asleep easily. That way, you will train yourself to become deeply relaxed whenever you do these movements. Then, if you awaken during the night, do not be concerned. Just do those same movements a few times more. You will regain your focus very quickly.

With a little practice you will become an expert at relaxing your body, calming your mind, and lulling yourself to sleep. When your sleep becomes easy and complete, you will be more alert and alive during waking hours. You will gain greater energy and vitality and enjoy a richer, more joyous life.

Mini-Move #2: Breath Surfing 2 (Going Deeper)

Now that you know the basics of Breath Surfing, try this delightful variation. It has a unique and different rhythm that will usher you into a state of even deeper repose. You will find this Mini-Move especially helpful should you wake up during the night. If you do awaken, do not be concerned. Do not stir yourself. Simply lie quietly, practice a few rounds of this Mini-Move, and savor the physical sensation of your own living, breathing body. *Never mind* whether you fall into a deep sleep, meander from one dream to the next, or lie in quiet contemplation, resting and renewing your vital energies. Simply surrender to those dreamy, drowsy sensations and think of nothing in particular. That will ensure that you get all the rest you possibly can and greet the new day with renewed energy and optimism.

Step 1. *Get comfortable.* Lie on your back in bed, or on a soft mat or carpet on the floor. You can use a pillow to support your head and neck if you like. Do whatever you need to get comfortable.

Take a few moments to check in with yourself. How does it feel to lie still like that? Do you feel relaxed and at ease, or restless? Drowsy or lucidly alert?

Are your eyes at rest, or do they move about? How do you breathe? Does your breathing feel light, easy, slow, and soft? Or do you tend to hold your breath? Is your breathing hurried or forceful?

Whatever you discover, just acknowledge it and let it be. Don't try to change anything at this point.

Step 2. *Home position.* Now please bring your fingertips to your sternum, or breastbone, just as you did in Breath Surfing 1.

The tips of your fingers rest lightly on your sternum, and your thumbs rest comfortably anywhere on your chest. Your elbows may lie on the bed or floor, or they may rest against your ribs. Let your wrists, hands, and fingers be at ease. Do not press. No force is required. Take a few moments to rest quietly like that.

Direct your attention to the movements of your breath. Each time you inhale, your chest rises and your thumbs rise with it. Each time you exhale, your chest sinks and your thumbs sink with it. Continue for six, seven, or more complete breath cycles.

Step 3. *Observe the movements of your right thumb.* Let the breath come and go of its own accord. Don't hurry. Take all the time you need for each breath.

As you breathe, direct your attention to your *right* thumb. Each time you inhale, your chest rises, and your thumb rises with it. Each time you exhale, your chest sinks and your thumb sinks with it. Continue for six, seven, or more complete breath cycles.

Step 4. *Go right.* Now, each time you slowly inhale, very gradually lift your right thumb a little bit. Then slowly exhale, relax your thumb, and allow it to return to your chest. Repeat the movement six, seven, or more times as desired.

Synchronize your movements with your breath. Little by little, your mind and your thoughts become synchronized with the slow, natural rhythm of the breath. Attend only to this breath, this movement, this moment.

Step 5. *Stop, rest, and feel.* Rest quietly for six, seven, or more complete breath cycles. Make no effort to breathe deeply or any special way. Notice the gentle rising and falling of your chest as you breathe. Does the right side of your chest feel different from the left?

Step 6. *Observe the movements of the left thumb.* Don't hurry. Let your breathing be light, easy, soft, and slow. As you breathe, direct your attention to your *left* thumb. Each time you inhale, your chest rises and your thumb rises with it. Each time you exhale, your chest sinks and your thumb sinks with it. Continue for six, seven, or more complete breath cycles.

Step 7. *Go left.* This time, each time you slowly inhale, very gradually lift your *left* thumb a little bit. Then slowly exhale, relax your thumb, and allow it to return to your chest. Repeat the movement six, seven, or more times as desired.

Notice how your chest moves when you lift your left thumb. Does one side of your chest move a little more freely, a little more fully? Make no effort to breathe deeply or any special way. Simply observe the natural variation of the breath, if any, in response to the movements of your thumb.

Step 8. *Stop, rest, and feel.* Rest quietly for six, seven, or more complete breath cycles. Allow your breath to come and go of its own accord. Notice the gentle rising and falling of your chest as you breathe now. Does the left side of your chest feel different now? Is your breathing a little freer, or fuller? When the breath is truly free, your mind and body become spacious, and the simple act of breathing in and breathing out becomes exquisitely pleasurable.

Step 9. *Go right and left.* Now we'll alternate the movements of the thumbs in a repeating two-breath sequence. Let's take it one breath at a time.

First breath: Slowly inhale and lift your *right* thumb. Slowly exhale, and lower your thumb. Notice how your chest moves. Does one side of your chest seem to move a little more freely?

Second breath: Slowly inhale and lift your *left* thumb. Slowly exhale, lower your thumb. Notice how your chest moves now. What do you feel?

To conclude: Repeat the above sequence three or four times, then rest for three or more complete breath cycles.

Notice how it feels to breathe now. When your breathing is easy, light, and natural, simply inhaling and exhaling is a pleasure. Your breath acts like an internal communication network, broadcasting calming, pleasurable messages to every cell of your body. This silent network of tranquility reaches billions of listeners!

Step 10. *Go deeper.* This next movement consists of a repeating three-breath sequence followed by a rest period. Again, let's take it one breath at a time.

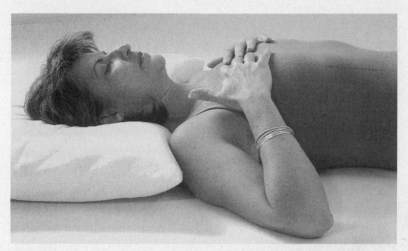

GO DEEPER 1. Slowly inhale and gradually lift your right thumb. Slowly exhale, and relax.

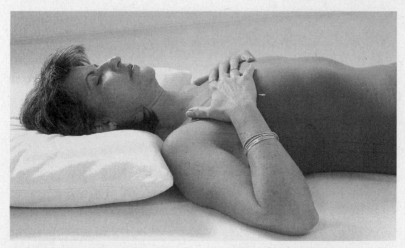

GO DEEPER 2. Slowly inhale and slowly exhale, doing nothing with your thumbs. Simply observe the rising and falling movement of your breath.

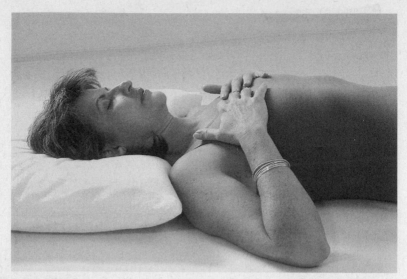

GO DEEPER 3. Slowly inhale, and gradually lift your left thumb. Slowly exhale, and relax.

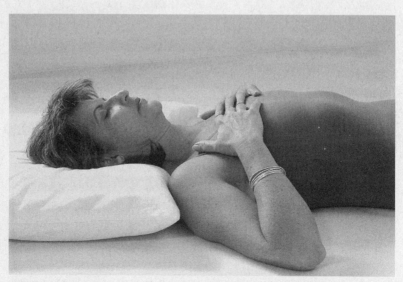

GO DEEPER 4. Rest quietly for three complete breath cycles.

First breath: Slowly inhale, and gradually lift your *right* thumb. Slowly exhale, and gradually lower your thumb. Synchronize the movement with your breath.

Second breath: Slowly inhale, and do nothing with your thumbs. Simply attend to your breath. Your chest rises and falls, and your thumbs rise and fall with it.

Third breath: Slowly inhale, and gradually lift your *left* thumb. Slowly exhale, and gradually lower your thumb. Allow your breath to subside completely.

To conclude: Rest quietly for *three* complete breath cycles. While you rest, continue to attend to the gentle rising and falling movements of your chest and your thumbs.

Continue, repeating the entire three-breath sequence plus the concluding rest period. On the first repetition, increase the rest period from three breaths to four. On the second repetition, increase it to five complete breath cycles. Continue like that, allowing the rest periods to get longer and longer. If you drift off or lose count, start over at the beginning.

You can continue in that way, gradually making the rest periods longer and longer. Make no effort to fall asleep. Simply allow the inner wisdom of your own mind and body to decide what happens next. Eventually, those prolonged periods of quiet rest will merge into a vast expanse of dreaming, drifting, and dozing, and the warm luxury of slumber will come to enfold you.

Variations:

1. Do any or all of this Mini-Move as indicated, but instead of lifting your thumbs, merely *lighten* them.
2. Do the movements of the thumbs in your imagination only. After a few rounds with the thumbs, try the index, middle, ring, and little fingers in turn.

3. Do this Mini-Move with your hands on the lower or middle breathing space. See what you discover!

Your own intelligence and intuition are your surest guides to finding the variation that works best for you.

Lulling Mini-Move #3: Rocking the Cradle

> O goddess, the slow swaying of a person's body
> whether by a moving vehicle or by self-induced movement
> calms her mental state so that she attains timeless
> wisdom and the bliss of transcendental consciousness.
>
> —VIJNANABHAIRAVA, *verse 83*

Have you ever sat quietly in a rowboat on a lake, simply letting the gentle rocking of the waves transport you into a state of deep relaxation and inner peace? Perhaps you have whiled away a balmy Sunday afternoon drifting, dreaming, and dozing in a rocking chair, a porch glider, or a hammock. As a child, you may remember being sweetly rocked to sleep in the arms of a parent or other caregiver.

If so, then you already know the power of gentle, rhythmic, rocking movements to soothe, to salve, to heal, and to lull. The lulling effect of rhythmic, rocking movement has been acknowledged in every land throughout the ages. There is a wonderful scene in book XIII of *The Odyssey* in which Odysseus, exhausted from years of war and privation, is lulled to sleep by the rhythmic movements of an oar-driven ship as it bounds over the waves. "But for that time he slept in peace, forgetful of all that he had suffered."

And of course, any American who lived through the '60s will remember the traditional rocker that was a fixture of President Kennedy's Oval Office. That was the president's favorite therapy for his war-torn back, and an all-purpose balm for the stress of what may well be the most stressful job in the world.

The medical profession also recognizes the salutary effects of gentle, sustained rhythmic rocking. A report in the *American Journal of Occupational Therapy* sums it up: "Rocking provides a general inhibitory or relaxing effect on the individual, thereby decreasing frustration, anxiety, tension, and/or blocking out an overstimulating environment." In other words, rocking is just the thing to gently lull you to sleep.

But don't worry, I'm not going to insist you run out and buy a rocking chair, a porch glider, or a rocking bed. There's really no need, because that same sort of gentle, lulling movement is available to you at this very moment. You can produce it with your own body anytime you feel the need. No equipment is required!

In fact, self-produced movement may be even more effective than the mechanical kind. I have discovered that the exquisitely gentle, rhythmic movements of your own body, especially when they are synchronized with the continuous, slow ebb and flow of the breath, are nature's safest, gentlest tranquilizer. They can help you overcome worry, fear, anxiety, tension, and stress, and bring you to a state of profound repose. And, as you are about to discover, they can also deliver you to the shores of sleep.

Note: This Mini-Move is presented in three parts. When you first practice this Mini-Move, please follow the instructions in the order given. Later, you can practice whichever movements give you the most peace. Remember, the Mini-Moves are for you. Please use them in the way that best suits your needs.

PART ONE: ROCKING THE CRADLE "TO"

Step 1. *Observe yourself in repose.* Please lie on your back with your legs straight, on a soft mat or carpet on the floor or in bed. Place your arms anywhere you like. Use a pillow to support your head if you feel the need. Make yourself as comfortable as possible.

- How does it feel to lie quietly like that? Notice how your body makes contact with the floor as you slowly, softly inhale and exhale. What parts of yourself touch the floor most distinctly? Is it your heels? Your buttocks? Some part of your back or shoulders?

- Turn your attention for a moment to your lower back—the part of your back that's just above your waist. Does your lower back lie in close contact with the floor, or is there a space between your lower back and the floor? Don't worry, this is not a test, and there is no right or wrong answer. Just see if you can feel what is the relationship between your lower back and the floor. You may even touch with your fingertips on either side of your lower back to help you feel.

- For some people, the lower back forms a kind of arch, leaving a considerable space between the lower back and the floor. For others, the lower back lies close to the floor, or in direct contact with it. Neither one is right or wrong—they are just different. For our purposes, it is enough simply to know how your own back lies in relation to the floor, without comparing, without judgment. Don't try to change anything. Just see how it is for you.

- Rest a little, allowing your breathing to be soft and slow. What parts of your body move as you breathe? If you were going to really allow your whole self to just sink into the floor, would you feel most able to do that while you were breathing in or breathing out?

Step 2. *Home position.* Please bend your knees and put the soles of your feet flat on the floor. Place your feet in such a way that you can hold your legs in this position easily, without excessive effort. You can try placing your feet a little closer or farther apart, a little closer or farther away from yourself. Whatever feels easy and comfortable for you, that's just right.

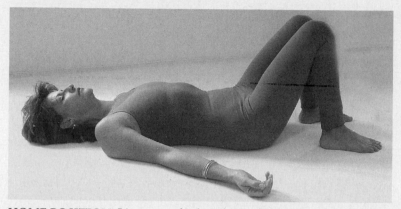

HOME POSITION. Lie on your back with your knees bent and your feet standing flat on the floor.

Step 3. *Push away.* Now, slowly inhale and as you do so, think of beginning to straighten your legs very gradually. The soles of your feet will push against the floor a little, as if you were going to

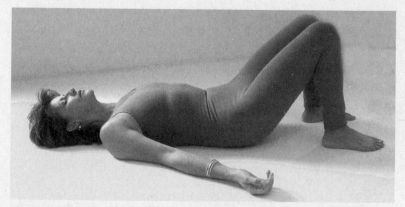

PUSH AWAY. Slowly inhale, and as you do so, think of extending your legs. Apply gentle traction to the floor, as if you were pushing away from you. Slowly exhale, and relax.

straighten your legs, but your knees remain bent, your feet stay right where they are. You apply a gentle traction against the floor with the soles of your feet.

Then, as you slowly exhale, gradually cease the effort and allow your legs to relax. The knees remain bent, the soles of your feet are flat on the floor.

- Repeat that movement several times, synchronizing your movements with your breathing. That means, however long it takes you to inhale, that's how long it takes you to gradually mobilize the muscles of your legs to apply that gentle push against the floor with the soles of your feet. However long it takes you to slowly exhale, that's how long it takes you to gradually relinquish the pressure, allowing the soles of your feet to rest on the floor as before. There's no apparent movement of your legs. They neither bend nor straighten, they just make a gentle, pulsating movement.

- You may find that when you push the soles of your feet like that on the floor, other parts of your body move as well. See if you can feel how as you inhale and press the floor, your hips move, too. Do they rock a little bit in a certain direction?

Inhale, push the floor with your feet, and simply allow your hips to rock of their own accord. You don't have to do anything; just let it happen. When your hips rock that way, does your lower back come closer to the floor or go farther away? Exhale, and relax. Your lower back returns to its neutral position.

- As in all of these Mini-Moves, make the movements light and easy. For our purposes, light, easy movements are more effective than big, forceful ones.

- Light, easy movements allow you to feel more accurately how you move, and how that movement affects your mind and body. Throughout this program, you are being guided to use your own senses, your own ability to feel, as a tool for self-healing.

Step 4. *Stop, rest, and feel.* Straighten your legs, and rest quietly for several complete breath cycles. Take a few minutes to feel the result of what you have done.

PART TWO: ROCKING THE CRADLE "FRO"

Step 5. *Draw your feet toward you.* Bend your knees and put your feet standing as before. Slowly inhale, and *think* of drawing your feet a little bit *toward* you. It's as if you were going to slide your feet

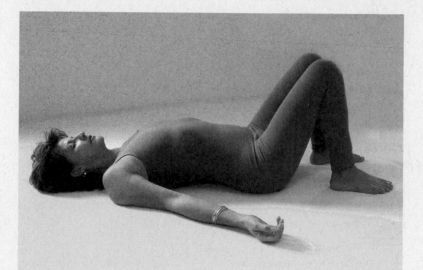

DRAW YOUR FEET TOWARD YOU. Slowly inhale, and *think* of drawing your feet a little bit *toward* you. Slowly exhale, and relax.

along the floor, closer to your bottom. But there is no apparent movement of your feet. Rather, the effort is so minimal that your feet remain in place. Very little force is required; you exert a very gentle traction against the floor, as if you were pulling it toward you. Then, slowly exhale, gradually relinquish the effort, and allow your feet to rest quietly on the floor. Again—slowly inhale, draw your feet toward you; slowly exhale, and relax.

- You will find that when you draw your feet toward you like that, other parts of your body move as well. See if you can feel how, as you inhale and draw your feet toward you, your hips move, too. They rock a little bit in a certain direction. What other parts of yourself move when you draw in your feet? Your back? Your chest? Your head?
- Inhale, draw your feet toward you, and allow your hips to rock a little bit. Exhale, gradually relax. When your hips rock to and fro like that, does your lower back lift up, away from the floor, or does it sink down closer to the floor?
- If this movement of the hips is unclear to you, you may wish to review "Pelvic Rock" in chapter 3. It will be helpful to you.

Step 6. *Stop, rest, and feel.* Straighten your legs, and rest. Feel the result of what you have done.

- Rest quietly and enjoy the stillness you've created within yourself. With just a few moments of synchronized movements and breathing, your mind and body become very still, and the volume of your thoughts is considerably reduced. Your mind is focused on this breath, this movement, this moment. The past and future recede from your awareness, and the present moment is the only reality.

PART THREE: ROCKING THE CRADLE TO AND FRO

Step 7. *Join the two movements.* Now we'll join the two moves we've done into a single, continuous action. Slowly inhale, and as you do so, gently, gradually push the soles of your feet away. Your hips rock and your lower back moves in that certain direction. Slowly exhale, and gradually stop pushing. Your hips and lower back return to neutral.

Then, slowly inhale again, and as you do so, gradually draw your feet toward you. Your hips rock in the opposite direction, and your lower back moves accordingly. Slowly exhale, and gradually allow your feet to rest on the floor. Your hips and lower back return to neutral.

Continue like that, alternating between one movement and the other. First you inhale and think of straightening your legs, pushing your feet away from you. Slowly exhale, relax. Then, inhale and think of bending your knees as if to draw your feet toward you. Slowly exhale, and relax. Repeat several times.

As you alternately push and draw your feet like that, notice the gentle, continuous, back-and-forth movement of your hips. With one breath your hips rock forward, and with the next breath they rock back. You may notice other parts of your body moving, too. The gentle oscillations of your feet, legs, and hips travel like a wave through your whole frame—through your ribs, your chest, your back, and your neck. You may even notice that your head rocks forward and back a little too. Don't try to make anything happen—just see what you discover.

Step 8. *Stop, rest, and feel.* Rest quietly for several complete breath cycles. The more, and longer, you rest between the movements, the better results you'll achieve.

- After you've completed a series of movements, rest quietly, giving your mind and body the time they need to regain full

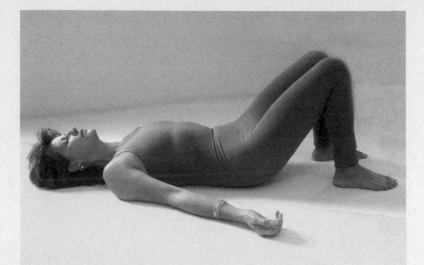

ROCK TO AND FRO. On the first breath, slowly inhale, push your feet away. Slowly exhale, and relax.

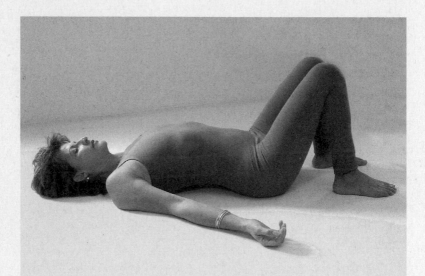

ROCK TO AND FRO. On the second breath, slowly inhale, draw your feet toward you. Slowly exhale, and relax.

strength, energy, and vitality. Allow the innate wisdom of your own mind and body to guide you to a state of deeply healing inner peace.

Application. Once you've practiced this Mini-Move a few times by day, you can try it at bedtime, right in bed. You won't need to run through the whole process step by step. Just do whatever movements you recall, whatever feels best to you. The gently synchronized movements and breathing will deliver you to the shores of sleep.

Lulling Mini-Move #4: Tongue in Cheek

An organic which lengthens by contracting clearly merits its own science.

—G. COULY

Our mouths are busy, busy, busy right from the first day of life. Nursing at the breast or bottle; discovering the world around us; exploring our own bodies; wordlessly vocalizing. These provide full-time occupation for our jaws, lips, and tongue during the first months. Later, discovering our favorite foods and eventually speaking—one of the crowning achievements of the human body and mind—keep us in a state of continual oral activity during waking hours.

Recent research reveals that our tongues get quite a workout during sleep, too. You heard earlier about the rapid eye movement, or REM, stage of sleep. Well, a recent study reveals that the tongue does its own peculiar dance during REM sleep, as well. Why? No one knows.

What we do know is that the jaw, lips, and tongue have a very intimate relationship with the brain. The exquisitely coordinated movements necessary for eating, facial expression, and speech require lots of brainpower, so the neural connection between the mouth and the brain is decidedly "broadband."

Generally speaking, the brain controls the body and its movements. It may surprise you to know that the reverse can also be true. We can use our own bodily movements to effect changes in the state of our brain. The lips, tongue, and jaw—with their broadband connections to the brain—provide one of our most powerful tools for regulating the state of the brain and nervous system.

The Relaxing Mini-Move that follows will bring your jaw, lips, and tongue to a state of profound repose. When your jaw, lips, and tongue are in repose, your mind becomes very still, and your whole body tends to follow suit.

As a result, your tense muscles begin to surrender, bringing you pleasurable sensations in various parts of your body. You may experience a pleasantly dreamy, drowsy state of tranquility and inner ease. And those troubling thoughts that cloud your mind? You can simply let them float away, leaving an expanse of clear blue sky. If you're ready for a good night's sleep, just get under the covers and do a few of these easy, effortless movements. Then rest awhile. What happens next? Try it, and see for yourself!

Note: This Mini-Move is presented in four parts. For a brief practice, you may do one or two parts. For a longer practice, do all four in succession. Please use the Mini-Moves in any way you see fit. You are free to develop your own variations!

PART ONE: HOME POSITION

Step 1. *Get comfortable.* Lie on your back in bed or on a mat or rug on the floor. You may also do this Mini-Move while lying on your side if you like. The movements are the same.

Make yourself as comfortable as possible, using pillows to support your head and neck. Some people find it very comforting to place a rolled blanket or towel under their knees. It may relieve strain on your lower back.

Take a few moments just to feel how your body lies against the bed or floor. Do you feel calm and relaxed, or tense and anxious? Notice your face, your lips, your forehead, your jaw. Is there any unwanted tension there? Do you tend to clench your jaw or grind your teeth? You needn't change anything. Just observe what is.

What parts of your body make the firmest contact with the bed or floor? Is it your feet? Your knees? Your buttocks or hip? Notice how your head rests against the bed or floor.

When you are resting quietly like that, where does your tongue come to rest in your mouth? Does it press against the back of your teeth, against the roof or the floor of your mouth? Don't try to change anything. Just observe what is.

Step 2. *Find the home position for the tongue.* Now gently touch the tip of your tongue to the inside of your right cheek, just to the

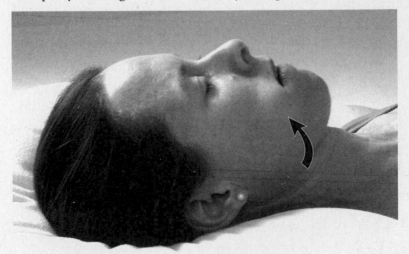

TONGUE IN CHEEK, HOME POSITION. Gently place the tip of your tongue at the inside of your right cheek, just to the right of the corner of your mouth.

right of the corner of your mouth, where your upper and lower lips meet. Your lips are together; your teeth are apart.

Now, with the tip of your tongue touching the inside of your cheek like that, slowly inhale. As you slowly inhale, very gently press your tongue outward against the inside of your cheek. It's as if you were exploring the cheek to determine its thickness, its texture, the degree of elasticity of the tissues there.

Slowly exhale, and as you exhale, gradually relax your tongue, allowing the pressure against the cheek to subside.

Pause a few moments if you like. Whenever you feel ready, try again. Slowly inhale, gently extend the tongue against the inside of the cheek. Slowly exhale, relax the tongue. And again, inhale, extend the tongue; exhale, and relax.

Please keep it all very light and easy. After all, this is done with tongue in cheek! So please, do give yourself permission to enjoy what you're doing. And don't worry! You are making all the right mistakes for learning.

Do several more movements like this. Here are some tips to help you get the best results.

- Synchronize the movement with your breathing. That means, however long it takes you to slowly inhale, that's how long it takes you to gradually extend your tongue. However long it takes you to slowly exhale, that's how long it takes you to relax your tongue.
- Press your tongue very gently and softly against the cheek. The moment you feel an increase in the resistance, that means you've done enough. The next time, do even less, so that the movement is lighter and easier than anything you can imagine.
- If you feel any discomfort in moving your tongue like this, please do the movement in your imagination only. Merely think the movement, but do nothing. For our purposes, imag-

inary movements are just as effective as real ones. Merely think the movement, and you will get all the benefits, effortlessly.

Step 3. *Stop, rest, and feel.* Enjoy the result of what you have done. Lie still, with your lips together, teeth apart. Let your breathing be easy, light, and free.

- As you rest quietly after those few gentle movements, you may notice that that your lips and tongue have become very still. Your tongue may come to rest in a different part of your mouth than it did before. Does it rest against the back of your teeth, against the roof your mouth, or somewhere else? Do you feel anything different about your jaw?

- You know, many of us tend to overwork the muscles of the jaw. We may clench the jaw or grind our teeth when we are under stress, or for no apparent reason, even during sleep. It's worth noting that the muscles of the jaw are considered part of the body's anti-gravity system, the muscles that support the body in standing upright. It may be that our excessively tense jaw muscles are one way that body and mind try to compensate for imbalances in the muscles of the neck, back, hips, legs, and feet. The good news is that inviting your jaw muscles to relax, as you are doing right now, can free up the other anti-gravity muscles, bringing you greater comfort, ease, and efficiency of movement.

PART TWO: THE UPPER POSITION

Step 4. *Lightly move the tip of your tongue to touch a spot just* above *the one you touched last time.* That's inside your cheek on the right side, near the juncture of your upper and lower lip, but this time it's just a touch higher than before. It's a difference of millimeters, not inches. Your lips are together, teeth apart. Your tongue goes between your teeth to press the inside of your cheek.

- Don't worry too much about the exact placement of your tongue: As long as the movements of your tongue remain easy and comfortable, you can't go wrong.

Now, with the tip of your tongue touching the inside of your cheek like that, a little higher than before, slowly inhale. As you slowly inhale, very gently press your tongue outward against the inside of your cheek.

- However long it takes you to slowly inhale, that's how long it takes you to gradually extend your tongue a little bit.
- As before, it's as if you were exploring the cheek to determine the quality of the tissues there. You may feel that the thickness, texture, and elasticity of the cheek are different at this new location.

Slowly exhale, and as you exhale, gradually relax your tongue, allowing the pressure against the cheek to subside.

- However long it takes you to slowly exhale, that's how long it takes you to gradually relax your tongue.

Continue. Slowly inhale, press the tongue against the inside of your cheek. Slowly exhale, relax your tongue. Repeat the gentle movement several times.

Slowly inhale, extend your tongue. Slowly exhale, and relax your tongue.

- If you feel any discomfort in moving your tongue like that, you may do the movement in your imagination only. Merely think the movements, but do nothing. For our purposes, imaginary movements are just as effective as real ones. Merely think the movement, and you will get all the benefits, effortlessly.

Step 5. *Stop, rest, and feel.* Allow your tongue to be completely at ease. Can you detect any changes in your jaw, your lips, your tongue? Does one side of your face feel wider, or more open? Can you feel that the muscles of your jaw, particularly on the right side, feel different from before? You may feel the sensation of gravity gently tugging your jaw back down toward the bed or floor. You may notice many other things that are unique to your own experience.

PART THREE: THE LOWER POSITION

Step 6. *Lightly move the tip of your tongue to touch a spot just* below *where you touched first time.* As before, it's inside your cheek on the right side, near the juncture of your upper and lower lips, but this time it's just a touch below the corner of the mouth. Lips together, teeth apart.

Now, with the tip of your tongue touching the inside of your cheek like that, slowly inhale. As you slowly inhale, very gently press your tongue outward against the inside of your cheek.

- As before, it's as if you were exploring the cheek to determine the quality of the tissues there. You may feel that the thickness, texture, and elasticity of the cheek are different at this new spot.

Slowly exhale, and as you exhale, gradually relax your tongue, allowing the pressure against the cheek to subside. Repeat the gentle movement several times.

Step 7. *Stop, rest, and feel.*

PART FOUR: FARTHER TO THE SIDE

Step 8. *Lightly move the tip of your tongue to touch a spot just* to the right *of where you touched the first time.* Again, it's inside your cheek on the right side, near the juncture of your upper and lower lips, but this time it's just a touch farther to the right of the corner of the mouth than it was before. Lips together, teeth apart.

Now, with the tip of your tongue touching the inside of your cheek like that, slowly inhale. As you slowly inhale, very gently press your tongue outward against the inside of your cheek.

Slowly exhale, and as you exhale, gradually relax your tongue, allowing the pressure against the cheek to subside.

Repeat several times at your own pace. You can pause whenever you like, then begin again.

Step 9. *Stop, rest, and feel.* Rest quietly, breathe easy. Let your tongue be completely at ease. Notice where your tongue is resting in your mouth now. Notice the feeling in your jaw.

- When you practice this Mini-Move on your own, do just a few movements, then rest quietly for several minutes. The rest periods are just as important as the movements, perhaps more so. It is the alternating structure of slow, synchronized movements and breathing and periods of quiet rest that make these techniques so effective.

- As you become more absorbed in the movements, you can allow longer and longer rest periods. The longer you rest between the movements, the more receptive you will be to the gentle rhythms of your own inner self, softly lulling you toward a state of blissful, restorative slumber.

If you like, you can go ahead and do all the same movements on the left side of your cheek. Another variation is to press with the tongue while exhaling, rather than while inhaling. It creates a slightly different effect, which some people seem to prefer. Or you can continue to rest quietly, allowing yourself to constructively linger in that timeless state. The longer you linger, the deeper will be your repose.

Lulling Mini-Move #5: The Ziggurat

Now I lay me down to sleep . . .
—TRADITIONAL BEDTIME PRAYER

Gravity never sleeps. For that reason, simply standing on our own two feet is for us human beings a precarious balancing act. From the viewpoint of physics, the human form, with its high center of gravity and narrow base of support (just those two itty bitty feet!), is an inherently unstable structure. With every move we make, we need to instantaneously adapt ourselves to the force of gravity, which relentlessly tries to drag us down.

Fortunately, the human body has something called an "anti-gravity system" that enables us to live happily and productively in this gravity-dominated world. The anti-gravity system is our automated postural-control system, and it's standard equipment for all healthy human bodies. It comprises the supporting muscles of the feet, legs, hips, back, and neck, as well as the neural mechanisms that control them. Whenever we sit or stand, it maintains the delicate balance of our upright posture with wondrous efficiency. That's what keeps us from falling down.

Even though we may not be aware of it, the simple act of standing upright requires a lot of muscular work and a lot of brain activity. Whenever we're sitting or standing, the anti-gravity system is on duty, ceaselessly vigilant in its efforts to keep us upright.

When we lie down, however, it's a whole different story. Lying down fundamentally alters our body's relationship with gravity. Instead of an unstable object with a high center of gravity and a narrow base, the body becomes a stable object with a low center of gravity and a broad base. No longer in constant danger of falling down, it *is* down, and no input is required to keep it that way.

Since it's not needed when we're lying down, the anti-gravity system takes a rest and the postural muscles relax. This global reduction in muscle activity reduces the excitatory impulses passing from the muscle nerves to the brainstem, setting the scene for rest, relaxation, and sleep.

At least, that's the ideal. Often, the reality is that the anti-gravity system keeps working at a lower pitch, even though we're lying still with our eyes closed. In that case, the anti-gravity muscles, especially those of the back and neck, keep sending excitatory signals to the brainstem, thereby delaying the onset of sleep. The purpose of this Mini-Move is to get those overactive anti-gravity muscles to quiet down so you can rest and sleep.

Why "the Ziggurat"? A *ziggurat* is a stepped pyramid. The step-like movements of this Mini-Move remind me of a ziggurat. Hence the name.

Note: This sleep-inducing Mini-Move employs movements that were presented in detail in Lengthening One Side in chapter 3 and Making Room in chapter 4. If any of the movements described here seem unfamiliar, please review those two. Then you'll be able to do the Ziggurat with perfect ease and enjoyment.

Step 1. *Get comfortable.* Lie on your right side with your left leg on top of your right. Bend your hips and knees so your knees are in front of you. Place a pillow under your head so it is comfortably

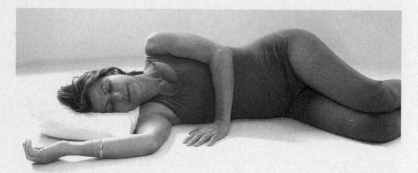

GET COMFORTABLE. Lie on your right side with your left leg on top of your right. Bend your hips and knees so your knees are in front of you.

supported. You may also wish to place a small pillow or a folded towel between your knees for greater comfort.

- If you prefer, you can do this exercise lying on your left side instead. You will get all the benefits.

Step 2. *Scan your body at rest.* Rest quietly for a few moments. See how it feels to lie like this. Notice how the side of your head, your cheek, and your jaw make contact with the pillow underneath you. Are they at ease?

- How does your right shoulder rest against the ground? How about the ribs on your right side? Do your shoulder and ribs rest firmly on the ground, or not? Can you feel any movement there, in your ribs, as you breathe?
- How about the right side of your waist? Does it completely surrender its weight to the ground, or not? Don't try to change anything. Just see what is.
- Feel the right side of your hip, your left thigh, your left knee, your left calf and ankle, your left foot. Which parts of yourself press the floor most distinctly when you are in repose?

Now, as you lie like that, simply observe the movements of your ribs on your *left* side. Each time you inhale, your ribs expand and your right shoulder and hip move a little to make room without any effort on your part. Each time you exhale, your ribs relax and your shoulder and your hip move back to their resting position.

Step 3. *Tip your hip down.* Slowly inhale, and as you do, gradually move your left hip *down*, away from your head, in the direction of your feet. It's as if your whole pelvis were rocking in the direction of your feet.

Then slowly exhale, and as you do, allow your hip to return to the resting position. The movement should be very small, with minimal force. That's all it takes.

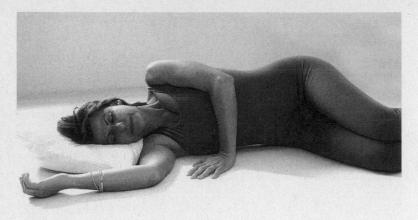

TIP YOUR HIP DOWN. Slowly inhale, and as you do, gradually tip your left hip *down,* away from your head, in the direction of your feet.

Rest for one or more complete breath cycles. Breathe easy, and see what you feel. Do you notice any difference in how your body lies against the floor now?

Repeat the movement several times. Slowly inhale, and tip your hip down. Slowly exhale, allow your hip to relax and return to its resting position. Rest and breathe after each movement.

- Make your movements light, easy, and slow. Remember, the less effort you expend, the more restful will be the result. Big, quick, powerful movements tend to be stimulating. Small, slow, gentle movements synchronized with breathing have a tranquilizing effect.
- Make no effort to breathe deeply or any special way. Simply let your breath come and go of its own accord. Don't huff and puff! Take all the time you need for each breath.

Each time you *inhale* and tip your hip down like that, what happens to your ribs and your waist on the right side of your body, underneath you? Do they seem to be lifting up away from the ground, or pressing closer down into it? Do your ribs and waist feel like they're resting on the floor more heavily, or are they getting a little lighter?

Each time you *exhale* and allow your hip to return to its resting position, what happens then? Do your ribs and your waist seem to be lifting up away from the ground, or pressing closer down into it? Do your ribs and waist feel like they're resting on the floor more firmly, or are they getting lighter?

Step 4. *Tip your hip in stages.* This movement is done in four stages. Each step is synchronized with one complete breath cycle.

Stage 1: Slowly inhale, and as you do, tip your left hip down a very small distance, perhaps one quarter of what you did in Step 2. Then, keeping your hip where it is, slowly exhale.

- You exhale, but do not allow your hip to come back to the resting position yet. Keep it *down*.

Stage 2: With your next breath, slowly inhale, and as you do, move your left hip down a little bit farther. Then, keeping your hip where it is, slowly exhale. Keep your hip where it is, a little farther *down* than in stage one.

Stage 3: With your third breath, slowly inhale and move your left hip still farther down. Then, keeping your hip where it is, slowly exhale. Keep your hip where it is, a little farther *down* than in stage two.

Stage 4: Now slowly inhale, keeping your hip where it is. Then slowly exhale and *very gradually* allow your right hip to relax and return to its natural resting position.

Step 5. *Stop, rest, and feel.* After you have done this four-stage movement *just once*, stop, rest, and feel for *three or more* complete breath cycles.

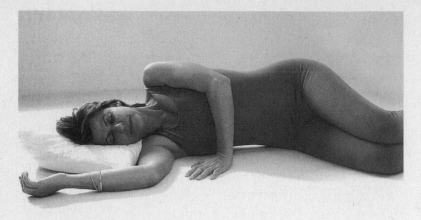

TIP YOUR HIP IN STAGES. On three successive breaths, tip your hip a little bit farther down and hold it there. With the final breath, slowly exhale and relax your hips completely. Your waist sinks into the floor.

What do you feel in your ribs and your waist on your right side now? You may feel them begin to press the floor a little more firmly than before. You may feel as if your waist is "sinking" into the floor. Either way, that means that your postural muscles are relinquishing their unnecessary effort and surrendering to the force of gravity. You are beginning to deeply relax.

- All physical movements, even very gentle ones like these, are stimulating and produce a feeling of physical excitation. When you rest quietly, you can feel those sensations gradually ebb away. Your body becomes very still and you feel tranquil.

By *taking time* to nurture this alternating ebb and flow of excitation, you are attuning yourself to the natural rhythm of action and repose as it is expressed in your own body. The more you become attuned to this rhythm, the easier it will be for you to rest and sleep.

You may repeat Steps 3 and 4 as desired. Rest frequently. The more time you take to rest between the movements, the more time your mind and body have to respond by becoming deeply relaxed. You are welcome to try the movements while lying on the other side, too.

If at any time you feel that sleepy, dreamy, drowsy feeling coming on, by all means surrender to it. Remember, the urge to sleep is a reflection of one of your body's most fundamental needs.

This Mini-Move is one of my personal favorites. I sometimes awaken an hour earlier than I want to. When I do, I just roll to my side and do a few rounds of the Ziggurat and go back to sleep. May it serve you as well as it does me.

Application. This Mini-Move can be done at bedtime, to help you fall asleep. If you awaken during the night or early morning, you may do it again. Remember, the rest periods between the movements are the most important part!

Lulling Mini-Move #6: Welcoming Sleep with Open Arms (Instead of Pacing the Floor)

> We are somewhat more ourselves in our sleeps; and the slumber of the body seems to be the waking of the soul.
> —SIR THOMAS BROWNE

In the event of insomnia, advises Deepak Chopra in his book *Restful Sleep*, "Don't give up, and don't get up." His thinking is that even if you're awake, you should stay in bed and rest. Lying quietly in bed is far more restful than pacing the floor, reading a book, or whatever else you might do at 4 a.m. Besides, if you're lying quietly in bed, you have a much better chance of drifting back to sleep than if you're vacuuming the living room, playing video games, or tweaking your PowerPoint presentation—activities that may end up making you even more wakeful than before.

In general, I endorse Dr. Chopra's approach, especially when used in conjunction with the lulling Mini-Moves presented here. If you wake up during the night, I encourage you to stay right where you are and practice any one of the lulling Mini-Moves you've learned so far. In most cases, they will bring you to a deeply restful state in which, whether you sleep or not, your body can renew its vital energies. That ensures that you will get all the rest you possibly can. Sleep on it!

However, there may be times when you become so wakeful, so restless and agitated, that to force yourself to lie quietly in bed would be agonizing. Anxiety attacks, excessive worry, and nightmares are just a few examples of things that can just about catapult you out of bed. Your muscles get tense, your heart races, and your breathing goes all out of whack. In that case, why punish yourself? Get out of bed for a while, and forget about sleep. Try something *different*.

The following techniques are designed to help you at those difficult times when you just can't keep yourself in bed. They are practiced in standing position. The idea is to do them until you become calm enough to comfortably return to bed. Once you're back in bed, you can do any other Mini-Moves in your favorite lying-down position. You already know how effective they can be.

The Mini-Move is presented in three parts for easy, effective learning. Each part teaches you something new about the movements of the breath. Once you've mastered the three parts in the order given, you may practice them separately, or as a single, complete sequence. Remember, the Mini-Moves are yours to use as you see fit.

PART ONE: ROLLING YOUR ARMS

Step 1. *Home position.* Stand with your feet parallel, your arms resting comfortably at your sides. Soften your focus and allow your eyelids to droop. Soften your gaze. Do not focus on anything in particular. As always, take all the time you need for each breath.

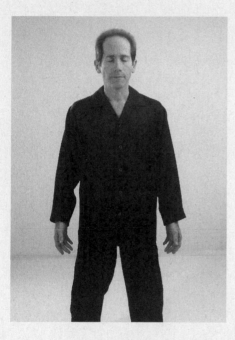

HOME POSITION. Stand with feet parallel, your arms resting comfortably at your sides.

Step 2. *Roll your arms outward.* Slowly inhale, and as you do, gradually rotate your arms outward so the palms of your hands face forward. Slowly exhale, relax your arms, and allow them to return to the home position. Repeat the movement five to ten times.

What is the path of the breath through your body when you move like that? Where is the feeling of fullness on inhalation? Is it in the back or the front of your body? Is it in the lower, middle, or upper breathing space?

ROLL YOUR ARMS OUTWARD. Slowly inhale and as you do, gradually rotate your arms outward so the palms of your hands face forward.

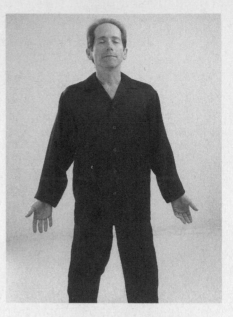

- Don't think where the breath *should* be; try to feel where it *is*. Using your intellect will lead you to confirm what you already know. Using your senses allows you to discover the new and unexpected.
- Synchronize your movements with your breath. However long it takes you to inhale, that's how long it takes to rotate your arms outward. However long it takes to exhale, that's how long it takes to bring your arms to the starting position.
- Each time you complete an exhalation, be sure to allow a moment's pause before the next inhalation begins. In that brief moment when your breath is empty, your mind becomes very still.

Step 3. *Rest and pause.* Slowly exhale and gradually allow the hands and arms to return to the starting position. Rest for at least three or more complete breath cycles.

See if there is any change in your breathing as a result of what you've done. Do you feel a little calmer, a little more at ease than before?

If you feel a little calmer, rest a little longer. If you feel agitated or anxious, you may continue to the next step now.

Step 4. *Roll your arms inward.* This time, slowly inhale and roll your arms *inward* so the palms of your hands face *behind* you. Then, slowly exhale, relax your arms, and allow them to return to the home position. Do not hurry. Take all the time you need for each breath.

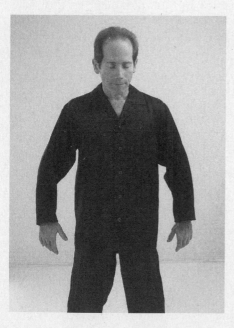

ROLL YOUR ARMS INWARD. Slowly inhale and roll your arms *inward* so the palms of your hands face *behind* you.

- What is the path of the breath through your body now? Where is the feeling of fullness on inhalation? Do you feel it in the front of your body or the back? Is it mostly in the lower, middle, or upper breathing space?

Repeat the movement five to ten times.

Step 5. *Rest and pause.* Slowly exhale and gradually allow the hands and arms to return to the starting position. Rest for at least three or more complete breath cycles.

Notice any changes in your mood, or your state of mind. If you feel peaceful and at ease, rest a little longer. If not, proceed to the next step now.

Step 6. *Roll your arms inward and outward.* Now you'll combine the two movements you've learned into a single, continuous, flowing action.

Slowly inhale and turn your arms outward so your palms face forward. Notice where the breath goes—what parts of yourself move as you breathe? Then slowly exhale and allow your arms to return to their starting position.

On the next breath, slowly inhale and turn your arms inward, so your palms face back. Where does the breath go? What parts of yourself move now? Then exhale and allow your arms to return to their starting position. Allow a moment's pause before the next inhalation begins. Repeat several times.

Step 7. *Stop, rest, and feel.* You may notice that you breathe more fully now. More parts of yourself are available to participate in the movements of respiration.

Do you feel a little calmer than when you began? If so, you may return to bed now. Otherwise, continue following the step-by-step instructions in the next section.

PART TWO: EXPANDING YOUR HANDS

Step 8. *Home position.* Stand quietly with your feet parallel. Your arms rest at your sides.

Step 9. *Spread the thumb and index finger.* Slowly inhale, and as you do, very gently spread the thumb and the index finger of each hand apart from each other. Then slowly exhale, and relax your hands.

The movement is a very gentle, gradual opening and closing of the hand at the thumb and index finger only. The rest of your hand remains still.

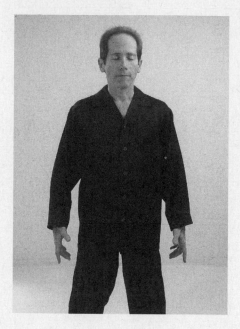

SPREAD THE THUMB AND INDEX FINGER. Slowly inhale, and as you do, very gently spread the thumb and the index finger of each hand apart from each other. Slowly exhale, and relax your hands.

Repeat that movement several times. Slowly inhale, spread the thumbs and index fingers apart. Slowly exhale, and relax.

• Where does your breath go when you move your hands like that? What parts of your body move as you breathe?

Step 10. *Spread the thumb and the little finger.* Slowly inhale, and as you do, very gently spread your thumbs apart from your little fingers and your little fingers apart from your thumbs. Then slowly exhale, and relax your hands. Don't hurry. Take all the time you need for each breath.

The movement is a gentle opening of the hand at the thumb and the little finger. The rest of the fingers remain still.

SPREAD THE THUMB AND THE LITTLE FINGER. Slowly inhale, and as you do, very gently spread your thumbs apart from your little fingers and your little fingers apart from your thumbs. Then slowly exhale, and relax your hands.

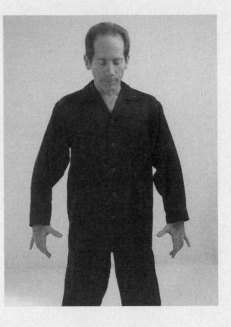

Repeat that movement several times. Slowly inhale, spread the thumbs and little fingers. Slowly exhale, and relax.

- Where does your breath go when you move your hands like that? What parts of your body move as you breathe?

Step. 11. *Combine the two movements.* Now you'll combine the two movements you've learned into a single, continuous, flowing action.

Slowly inhale and gently spread your *thumbs* and *index* *fingers* apart. Slowly exhale, relax. Take all the time you need between the end of your exhalation and the beginning of the next inhalation.

Whenever you're ready, begin the next inhalation. As you slowly inhale, spread your *thumbs* and your *little fingers* apart. Then slowly exhale, and relax. Repeat several times.

- Can you feel that the breath takes a different path through your body depending on whether you open the thumb/index or the thumb/little finger?

Step 12. *Stop, rest, and feel.* How does it feel to stand on your own two feet now? Do you feel more at ease than when you began? Do you feel a little more inclined to sleep? If so, you may return to bed now. Otherwise, continue following the step-by-step instructions in the next section.

PART THREE: WELCOMING SLEEP WITH OPEN ARMS

Step 13. *Welcome sleep with open arms.* Slowly inhale, and as you do, turn your arms outward so your palms face forward. At the same time, spread your thumbs apart from your index fingers. Slowly exhale, and allow the breath to subside completely.

Allow the next inhalation to come of its own accord. Then, slowly inhale, turn your arms inward so your palms face back, and spread your thumbs apart from your little fingers. Then slowly exhale, relax your arms, and relax your hands.

- Allow your breath to be guided by the movement and the movement, in turn, to be guided by the breath. Any changes will happen spontaneously, without any effort of will.

Step 14. *Stop, rest, and feel.*

WELCOME SLEEP WITH OPEN ARMS 1. Slowly inhale, and as you do, turn your arms outward so your palms face forward. At the same time, spread your thumbs apart from your index fingers. Slowly exhale, and relax.

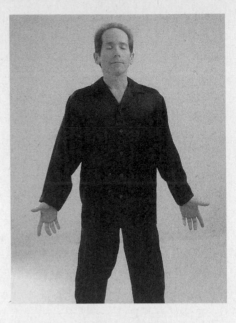

WELCOME SLEEP WITH OPEN ARMS 2. Then slowly inhale, turn your arms inward so your palms face back, and spread your thumbs apart from your little fingers. Then slowly exhale, relax your arms, and relax your hands.

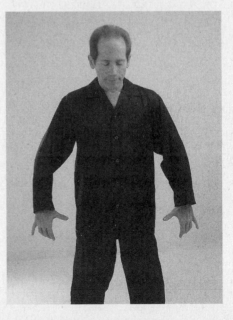

- As you rest, notice how it feels to breathe. Can you feel how this way of moving and breathing is helping to "make room" inside yourself? See what you discover.

- Breath is movement; without movement there is no breath. Just as each snowflake has its own unique pattern, so does each breath you take. Each breath finds its own unique path through your body, depending on the way you move as you breathe.

- By varying the movements of respiration, you open new pathways for the breath. Your body becomes spacious. Your breathing gets fuller and freer, and you feel more fully alive. It brings you pleasure and peace.

- When you are fully alive, sleep is never a problem. If you need sleep, you will sleep. When you awaken, you'll feel more alert and energetic all day long.

- Now that you have graciously welcomed sleep with open arms, you can lie down in bed and receive your guest. You may drift, you may dream, you may doze. By all means, follow your dream to its illogical conclusion. Soon enough you will lie warm in the gold of dawn.

The Rush to Sleep

In this fast-paced world of ours, most of us are rushing all the time. Rushing to go here or there, rushing to do this or that. And crazy as it sounds, we even *rush to sleep*!

Think about it: We set aside eight, or seven, or six hours for our nightly rest. Then we try to shoehorn all of our much-needed rest into that narrow little slipper of time. It's an awfully tight fit!

Sleeping on such a tight schedule produces lots of anxious anticipation. "Am I still awake? I have to be up at six! I don't have time to waste!" That kind of thinking can excite your mind and body, producing a flood of stress hormones that can delay the onset of sleep.

What can you do? Turn that bedtime *rush* hour into a bedtime *hush* hour! Here's how: If you need eight hours' sleep, allow yourself eight and a half or even nine hours in bed. That's right— get into bed thirty to sixty minutes earlier than you absolutely need to.

Do that, and the pressure is off. All you do is rest quietly, relax your body, clear your mind, and *think of nothing in particular*. Take all the time you need for each breath. You may drift, you may dream, you may doze, all at your own natural pace.

Give it a try. That luxurious "hush hour" really sets the scene for sounder sleep.

Mind Management

Clearly, what you do with your mind matters. And that's especially true when it comes to bedtime. For example, a psychological survey of pre-sleep thought patterns revealed that sound sleepers most often think of *nothing in particular*, whereas troubled sleepers think of things like jobs, taxes, and health concerns. The results suggest that troubling or overly stimulating thoughts can keep you awake. On the other hand, thinking of nothing in particular can help you get into just the right frame of mind for a restful night of dozing and dreaming.

When your mind is calm and clear of disturbing thoughts, it's much easier to quiet down and get ready to sleep. It's important to respect the integrity of your mental processes, however, and not try to *control* your mind. Your thoughts, emotions, and memories are your most reliable sources of information about yourself and the world around you. You don't want to distort or disrupt that natural information system!

Rather than mind-control strategies, I favor mind *management*. Mind management allows you to gently moderate your thought processes so you can adapt more effectively to whatever you're doing in the moment. When you're writing or speaking or performing any complex task, your mind should be alert and awake. You want to be able to process a wide variety of thoughts as quickly as possible. But when it's time to rest, you need to be able to shift your mental gears. Your thinking naturally slows down, and the volume of your thoughts is considerably reduced. Your mind becomes calm and clear.

The Mini-Moves excel at helping you achieve the calm, clear quality of mind that is most supportive of deep rest and sound sleep. Even so, there are some simple mind-management techniques that you may wish to use in conjunction with the Mini-Moves. You'll find these helpful at times when your mind is awash with stimulating thoughts, and you prefer to rest. Here are a few to try:

Nothing in particular. When it's time for bed, do as sound sleepers do: Set aside all mundane concerns, rest quietly, and think of nothing in particular.

Passing clouds. If and when troubling thoughts do arise, imagine that they are passing far over your head like fluffy white clouds in a clear blue sky. Just as clouds are vaporous forms in the sky, thoughts are vaporous forms in your mind. *Rest assured,* they have no power over you.

Turn on your "mental" radio. Imagine that your thoughts are being broadcast to you on a radio. Then, imagine that the radio is in another room, with the door ajar. You can hear the radio playing, but you can't quite make out the words.

If you are inclined to visual thinking, you can use an imaginary TV instead. Imagine that you are placing it just out of viewing range, so the picture is indistinct. The smaller the screen, the better. Imagining a black and white TV is good, too!

"Not now." Say silently to yourself, *"In this moment I choose quiet rest. Nothing else is required of me in this moment, only quiet rest and a calm, clear mind."* Once you have made that resolve, you may greet any intruding thoughts with the gentle yet firm statement, *"Not now!"*

You may use these gentle, non-intrusive mind-management techniques to calm and clear your mind at any time. They also make a great prelude to any of the lulling Mini-Moves presented in this chapter.

Sleep Continuity Versus Sleep Reversibility

Many people expect to get into bed and sleep *continuously* all night long, never waking up 'til morning. But that's an unrealistic expectation. The truth is that all human sleepers briefly wake up fifteen to thirty-five times a night. That's part of our natural sleep rhythm!

The difference between sound sleepers and troubled sleepers is not that sound sleepers sleep through the night and troubled sleepers wake up. The difference is this: *Sound* sleepers wake up those fifteen to thirty-five times, but they return to sleep quickly. Most of the time they don't even remember waking up. *Troubled* sleepers wake up and stay up. Therefore sound sleep depends not on *continuity*, but rather on *reversibility* of sleep. Reversibility of sleep means you can wake up, go back to sleep, wake up, and go back to sleep again, as needed.

The concept of reversible action was first articulated by Dr. Moshe Feldenkrais, the modern-day sage of mindful movement. In his groundbreaking book, *The Potent Self,* Feldenkrais wrote:

> Reversibility is a feature of all correct action, even sleep. Thus, the well-coordinated mature person, such as found among people who

have succeeded in making their occupation their pleasure, can go off to sleep when he feels like it and wake up when necessary. Moreover, all healthy animals and humans do not object to being awakened, as they can stop sleeping and resume sleeping without trouble. The ability to stop an action, a process, restart it, reverse it, or drop it all together is one of the finer criteria of proper *acture.* [Emphasis in original]

It is not necessary to explore the full implications of this passage. They are vast, not only for sleep but for all human action, for life in general. For our purposes, it's enough to note that Feldenkrais identified sleep as a paradigm case of reversibility, which he notes is a "feature of all correct action." I have recast this principle to make it more sleep-specific, as follows: *Reversibility is a feature of all natural, restful sleep.* I believe this more sleep-specific formulation is true to the spirit of the original.

When your sleep is not fully reversible, you feel that you can't trust yourself to recover from an unexpected awakening. Therefore, you dread being awakened, and you tend to resent anyone or anything that disturbs your slumber. That leads to something I call The "Oh, s--t!" Effect. When you wake up unexpectedly, the first thing you do is to say to yourself, "Oh, s--t!" (or a more genteel equivalent). Those two words are very powerful! They express your stubborn unwillingness to accept what already is—a foolproof recipe for frustration. That sets off a cascade of stressful reactions in your body. And, as we have seen, stressful reactions arouse you and make you far less likely to get back to sleep anytime soon.

Now here's the good news: Reversibility of sleep can be learned. The Mini-Moves presented in this chapter guide you step-by-step toward deep, restful, fully reversible sleep. For best results, practice every night at bedtime. Sleep will come to you sweetly, without any effort of will. If you awaken during the night, practice again. Little by little, you will merge back into that sleepy, dreamy, drowsy state. Practice often! The effect is cumulative. Eventually your sleep will become fully reversible. Your days will be sweeter and more livable, and each night will be a new opportunity to bask in the velvety shadows of sounder, more restful sleep.

Late-Night Awakenings: Burden or Blessing?

Many people complain of late-night or early-morning awakenings. Are you one of them? Do you wake up at 2 a.m., or later, and remain awake for forty-five minutes or an hour? Do you blame those wakeful periods for restless nights and drowsy, unproductive days?

In my work with troubled sleepers, I have sometimes found it helpful to consider the situation from another angle: Perhaps the problem is not the awakenings themselves, but our rigid expectations about sleep. Consider the following:

There is considerable evidence that in ancient times our ancestors slept in two shifts. They'd go to bed soon after sundown, then awaken for an hour or more after midnight. This so-called nightwatch could be a time of lucid waking rest, quiet contemplation or prayer, stoking the fire, tending to children or animals, or just gazing at the heavens. Then it was back to bed for a "second sleep" lasting 'til dawn. At that *leisurely pace*, our ancestors could easily enjoy all the restful sleep they needed between dusk and dawn.

Walt Whitman (1819–1892) celebrated the nightwatch in his poem "A Clear Midnight":

> This is thy hour O Soul, thy free flight into the wordless,
> Away from books, away from art, the day erased,
>   the lesson done,

Thee fully forth emerging, silent, grazing,
  pondering the themes thou lovest best,
Night, sleep, death, and the stars.

The nightwatch can be viewed as part of our ancestral sleep legacy, and a product of our natural bodily rhythms. It is also a source of spiritual sustenance and renewal—much needed in these turbulent times! Sadly, our *rush to sleep* often turns that natural, nourishing pause in the sleep process from ally to enemy.

As I write this, I have quite recently resettled in New Mexico, in the mountains east of Albuquerque. Last night, I attended a dinner party at the home of some new friends in Santa Fe, forty-five miles north of my home, and then spent the night with a colleague nearby. The party was wonderful, but, spurred on by the good company and general merriment, I ate more than I should have. I was in bed by midnight, and I slept soundly for a few hours. But at about 3 a.m. I was awakened by a disturbing dream and the rumblings of my own stomach. I was wide awake.

I slowly rolled out of bed and stood up, taking care not to open my eyes wide nor to focus very distinctly on any object, lest I become further aroused. For ten or fifteen minutes I practiced Welcoming Sleep with Open Arms. As I did that, I savored the silence and solitude of that late hour. I surrendered myself to the ultimate reality of "this breath, this movement, this moment." At one point, a few fragments of the just-cited Whitman poem meandered across my mind: "Night, sleep, death, and the stars." Little by little, the Mini-Moves delivered me to a state of profound peace and serenity.

I lay down on the bed and extinguished the light. I was in that sleepy, dreamy, drowsy state, neither fully awake nor quite asleep, that I have come to know so well. I did a few rounds of Breath Surfing. I remember feeling that this had been one of the deepest and most pleasurable meditations I had ever experienced. My next thought, whatever it may have been, was obscured by the softly falling velvet curtain of blackness. I rested peacefully until morning, sleeping a half hour longer than I had planned. In spite of the half-hour interruption in my sleep, I awoke refreshed and energized and feeling spiritually renewed. It was a beautiful, cool April day with deep blue, cloudless skies. I got into my car and drove home, exulting in the stunning mountain vistas of New Mexico's Route 14, the Turquoise Trail.

• Sleep on it. You may come to regard the nightwatch as a precious opportunity rather than an unwelcome interruption. Then simply allow yourself all the time you need in bed, all the time you need to let the natural sleep process unfold. That brings you deeper, more nurturing rest and a sweeter, more gracious relationship with your own body and spirit.

A Return to the Self: The Spiritual Dimension of Sleep

The Dalai Lama, interviewed in the *Utne Reader,* has called sleep our "[m]ost important meditation! . . . Not for nirvana, but for survival." His Holiness is quite right, of course—we wouldn't survive long without our daily dose of "vitamin S." But sleep is far more than just "survival meditation." It can also be a profound adjunct to any spiritual practice.

Between waking and sleeping lies a state of what the ancient yogic seers called the *nirvikalpa*, the state free of thought-constructs. Modern science calls this the hypnagogic state. This is our natural gateway to the wild interior of our minds. It is the common point of departure for meditation, introspection, contemplation, dreams, and *sleep.*

In truth, sleep is our nightly *return to the self,* whether we are aware of it or not. During waking hours everything we see, hear, feel, and *do* seems to draw us out of ourselves. Immersed and engaged in that outer world of people and things—of action—we forget what we *really* are. When we lie down to sleep, we withdraw our awareness from that tumultuous outer world. We go inside, to *be with ourselves,* in the moment. There, our hearts open to dreams and wonder, and we catch a nightly glimpse of our original self, unencumbered by the stresses and strains of daily life.

This lonely confrontation with self may be difficult for some. It may evoke feelings that we would prefer to ignore. But for those of us who are inclined to introspection, it is a great gift. At that moment of stillness, we return to our source in nature and the cosmos, we surrender to a power greater than ourselves, and the attitude of prayer and meditation comes to us spontaneously, without any effort of will.

This restful path to higher consciousness was well traveled by the yogis of ages past. For example, verse 75 of *Vijnanabhairava* (*Divine Consciousness*), a millennium-old manual of yogic meditation practices, advises:

> When you are about to fall asleep
> and all external objects have faded from view,
> concentrate on the state between sleep and waking.
> There the Supreme Goddess will reveal herself.

In modern times, great scientists and artists have looked to the hypnagogic state as a font of creative inspiration. Einstein realized an important piece of his relativity theory while strolling on a sunbeam, deep in a dream. Kekule identified the circular structure of the benzene atom while dreaming of teeming serpents. Vincent van Gogh used to say that the pictures came to him "as if in a dream." And the great conductor Arturo Toscanini used to enter the hypnagogic state during his concerts, as revealed in a recently published letter:

> Do you know that at the modulation of E flat [in the Adagio of Beethoven's Ninth] I always conduct with my eyes closed? I see extremely bright lights far, far away; I see shadows moving around, penetrated by rays that make them even more disembodied; I see flowers of the most charming shapes and colours. And the very music I'm conducting seems to descend from up there—I don't know where!

So you see, that time you spend each night waiting for the ferry to Slumber Land need not be wasted. It can be a time of deep introspection and a rich source of insight. In that case, you can enjoy the seeming paradox that for you, *sleep* will become a vehicle for *self-awakening*.

Appendix A

* * * *

For Further Exploration

Sounder Sleep Sominars
Phone: 866-864-4071
Web site: www.soundersleep.com

This is the official Web site of the Sounder Sleep System. It includes a current schedule of public programs and professional training opportunities; online marketplace for Sounder Sleep media; directory of authorized instructors in North America and Europe, plus information and published articles on the system.

The Feldenkrais Guild® of North America
3611 SW Hood Avenue, Suite 100
Portland, OR 97239
Phone: 800-775-2118
E-mail: guild@feldenkrais.com
Web site: www.feldenkrais.com

The primary source for information about the Feldenkrais Method of movement education. Web site includes informational materials; directory of teachers; list of professional training pro-grams; online bookstore, and more.

Feldenkrais Resources
830 Bancroft Way, Suite 112
Berkeley, CA 94710
Phone: 800-765-1907 or 510-540-7600
E-mail: Feldenres@aol.com
Web site: www.feldenkraisresources.com

Feldenkrais Resources carries a wide selection of books, audio, and video on the Feldenkrais Method and related fields of move-ment education. They also offer regular classes and professional training in the Feldenkrais Method at their Berkeley location, and elsewhere. Their excellent printed catalog comes out every two years.

Appendix B

★ ★ ★
★

Mini–Moves in Brief

The Mini-Moves as presented in chapters 3 through 5 have been carefully composed to give you a guided, step-by-step learning experience similar to what you'd receive in one of my Sounder Sleep Sominars. They will enable you to learn in depth, practice effectively, and achieve the most satisfying possible results.

Once you have familiarized yourself with a Mini-Move in its expanded form, you may use the brief synopsis below as an aid to further practice. The synopses contain only the principal movements. *They are intended only as an aid to practice and memory, not as a substitute for the full text.*

Chapter 3

Relaxing Mini-Move #1: The Pelvic Rock

1. *Home position.* Lie on your back and rest quietly for several minutes. Notice which parts of your body make contact with the floor. Bend your knees and put your feet standing, with the soles of your feet flat on the floor.
2. *Tilt your hips back.* Very gently and slowly, tilt your hips a little bit so that the lowermost tip of your tailbone lifts

upward, toward the sky, and your waist and lower back move downward, toward the earth. Then relax. Repeat several times, then rest.

3. *Tilt your hips forward.* This time, slowly and gently tilt your hips the other way. The lowermost tip of your tailbone moves down, toward the earth, and your waist and lower back lift up, away from the floor. Then relax. Repeat several times, then rest.

4. *Tilt your hips forward and back.* Slowly tilt your hips forward, then tilt them back. Repeat several times, then rest.

5. *Rhythmic pulsation.* Tilt your hips forward and back with very small, very quick motions. The gentle, rocking motion of your hips generates a pulsation that spreads through your entire frame. Continue as long as desired. Then rest.

Relaxing Mini-Move #2: Unlocking Your Rib "Cage"

1. *Observe yourself in action.* Stand, and gently turn and look to the right and to the left several times. Make a mental note of some object that you can see to your far right, and another to your far left.

2. *Float your shoulder.* Lie down. Slowly, gently lift your right shoulder a little bit off the floor. Then gradually allow your shoulder to sink back to the floor. Repeat several times, then rest.

3. *Synchronize your head and shoulder.* Each time you float your right shoulder upward, deliberately roll your head very gently to the left. Repeat several times, then rest.

4. *Unlock your "cage."* Slowly float your right shoulder upward, and as you do so, *very gently* press your left shoulder into the floor. You needn't press hard! Then lower your right shoulder, and stop pressing with the left. Repeat several times, then rest.

5. *Side two.* Repeat Steps 2 through 4 on the other side.

6. *Rhythmic turning.* Turn your trunk right and left, and allow your arms to swing freely. Allow your chest to be free and flexible. Look for the most pleasurable way to do the movement, so it feels really delicious.

Relaxing Mini-Move #3: Lengthening One Side of Your Trunk

1. *Raise your arms.* Stand up, and slowly raise your right arm to the ceiling without strain, without stretching. Now do the same with your left arm. How does that feel? Make a mental note of it so you'll have something to compare with later on.

2. *Observe yourself in repose.* Lie on your back for a few moments. Notice how the various parts of your body make contact with the floor underneath you.

3. *Home position.* Lie on your right side on a soft rug, a blanket, or an exercise mat on the floor. Bend your legs at the hip and knee so that your knees lie on the floor in front of you. The left leg lies on top of the right in a symmetrical fashion.

4. *Slide your foot down.* Now slide your left foot a little bit down, away from your head, as if you were going to straighten your leg.

5. *Mobilize your shoulder.* Lie on your right side, as in step 3. Very gently move your left shoulder up, in the direction of your ear.

6. *Move your hip down.* Without moving your foot or leg, can you move your hip down, away from your shoulder?

7. *Elongate your leg.* Straighten your left leg and move your left heel downward, away from your head, so that your leg gets *longer.*

8. *Lengthen one side.* Lie on your right side in the Home Position. Very gently, move your left hip down, and at the same

time move your left shoulder up, toward your ear. Your shoulder and your hip move apart, and the whole left side of your body grows longer.

9. *Feel the difference.* Slowly roll to your side and stand up and see how it feels. Slowly raise your left arm toward the ceiling. How does that feel now? Try raising your right arm. Which arm feels lighter, longer? Which arm is easier to raise?

10. *Explore the other side.* Lie down and rest for a while. Then, when you're ready, lie on your right side, and repeat all the movements, this time with your left hip and shoulder. Don't hurry. Take your time, and see what you discover.

Relaxing Mini-Move #4: Slouch and Recover

1. *Observe your sitting posture.* Sit on the front half of the seat, any way that you like as long as you are not leaning on the backrest. Notice how it feels to sit like that.

2. *Look down.* Slowly lower your head and look down to see your belt buckle. Slowly raise your head, and sit up. Repeat several times, then rest.

3. *Engage your ribs and chest.* Each time you lower your head and eyes to look down, your chest tends to tip downward, toward your belly. As you raise your head and eyes, your chest rises to help bring the head to the upright position. Repeat several times, then rest. (Place your fingertips on your sternum if you like.)

4. *Engage your lower back.* (Place your hand on your lower back if you like.) Each time you slouch, allow your lower back to move backward. Your back rounds slightly. Each time you recover, allow your lower back to move forward. Repeat several times, then rest.

5. *Rock your pelvis.* Lowering your head produces a gentle backward rocking of your pelvis; you sit more on the *rear-*

ward portion of your buttocks. Raising your head produces a gentle forward rocking of your pelvis; you sit more on the *forward* portion of your buttocks. Repeat several times, then rest.

6. *Put it all together.* Rock forward and back several times, engaging the head and eyes, chest, and lower back.

7. *Observe your seated posture.* See if there is any difference, however small, in the way that you sit now, as compared to when you began.

Relaxing Mini-Move #5: Painting the Air (Freeing Your Arms for Action)

1. *Raise your arms.* Slowly raise both arms in front of you, as if you were reaching for your keyboard, and slowly lower your arms to your knees again. Do your arms feel light and easy to move, or heavy and cumbersome? Repeat several times, then rest.

2. *Raise your arms while slouching.* Slouch as you learned to do in the previous Mini-Move. While slouched, slowly raise your arms and lower them several times in succession. Remain slouched the entire time you're moving your arms. Repeat several times, then rest.

3. *Raise your arms while sitting up tall.* Sit as tall as possible without strain. While holding your body upright like that, slowly raise and lower your arms several times. Repeat several times, then rest.

4. *Synchronize your arms with your trunk.* To begin, slouch. Then as you recover from the slouch and come to sit up tall, slowly lift your arms. Then gradually slouch again, and slowly lower your arms. Synchronize the movement of your arms with the movements of your trunk. Repeat several times, then rest.

5. *Air-painting.* As you raise your arms, paint the imaginary canvas with the backs of your hands in an upward-sweeping brushstroke. As you reach the top of the stroke, gently allow your wrists to bend back so that the palm side of your hands faces the canvas. Then paint the canvas in a downward-sweeping stroke with the palms of your hands. Repeat several times, then rest.

6. *Advanced air-painting.* As you begin to stroke downward with your right hand, raise your left hand to stroke upward. When you have raised your left hand as far as you like and your right hand has returned to its starting position, lower your left hand as you raise your right. Repeat several times, then rest.

7. *Feel the difference.* Slowly raise your arms as if to reach the keys of a keyboard, and slowly lower them. See how it feels now. Do your arms feel light or heavy? Are they easy to move, or cumbersome?

Relaxing Mini-Move #6: To Banish Neck and Shoulder Tension: Hang Loose!

1. *Calibrate your shoulders.* Take note of the distance between the tip of your right shoulder and your right earlobe. Compare that with the distance between your left shoulder and your left earlobe.

2. *Calibrate your head and eyes.* Slowly and gently turn your head and eyes to the right and to the left, without straining. Does your head turn farther to one side or the other? Which feels freer and easier, turning to the right or the left?

3. *Raise your right shoulder.* As you slowly inhale, gently raise your right shoulder. Repeat several times, then rest.

4. *Raise the shoulder in three stages.* Slowly inhale and raise your shoulder about one-quarter of the way, and hold it there.

Slowly exhale. Repeat two more times, raising the shoulder higher each time. Then slowly inhale, and as you exhale, slowly lower the shoulder and relax. Repeat several times, then rest.

5. *Recalibrate your shoulder.* Take note of the distance between the tip of your right shoulder and your right earlobe now. Is it different than before?

6. *Recalibrate your head and eyes.* Slowly and gently turn your head and eyes to the right and to the left, without straining. Does your head turn farther to one side or the other? Which side feels freer and easier now, turning to the right or the left?

7. *Side two.* Repeat Steps 3 through 5 with the left shoulder.

Chapter 4

Calming Mini-Move #1: L.E.S.S. Is More

1. *Explore the lower breathing space.* Place your hands side by side, palms down, on your lower abdomen. As you slowly inhale, your belly rises and expands, and your hands move with your belly. As you slowly exhale, your belly sinks, and your hands sink with your belly. Your breath does the movement, not you.

2. *Explore the middle breathing space.* Place your right hand on the lowermost rib on the right, palm down, so that the rib is cradled in the crease of the palm of your hand. Place your left hand in the same position on the left side. As you slowly inhale, your ribs rise and expand, and your hands move with your ribs. As you slowly exhale, your ribs sink, and your hands sink with your ribs. Your breath does the movement, not you.

3. *Explore the upper breathing space.* Bring your hands to the upper part of your chest, below your collarbones and above

your breast. Arrange your hands so that the tips of your middle fingers lightly touch each other in the middle of your chest. As you slowly inhale, your chest rises and expands, and your hands move with your chest. As you slowly exhale, your chest sinks, and your hands sink with your chest. Your breath does the movement, not you.

Calming Mini-Move #2: Making Room

1. *Home position.* Lie on your right side on a bed or on a mat or carpet on the floor.
2. *Your ribs expand as you breathe.* As you slowly inhale, your ribs swell and expand. As you exhale, your ribs relax.
3. *Your shoulder moves as you breathe.* As you slowly inhale, see if you can detect any movement of your shoulder, no matter how small or subtle. As your ribs expand, they gently displace the shoulder to make room for their expansion.
4. *Your hip moves as you breathe.* As you slowly inhale, see if you can detect any movement of your hip, no matter how small or subtle. As your ribs expand, they gently displace your hip to make room.
5. *The side of your body lengthens as you breathe.* Each time you inhale, the whole side of your body grows longer. Each time you exhale, you deeply relax.

Calming Mini-Move #3: Things Are Looking Up!

1. *Get comfortable.* Sit in a chair or lie quietly on your back, and softly close your eyes. Notice the feeling in your lips, your cheeks, your forehead. Does your face feel at ease, or is it tense and contracted?
2. *Raise your eyebrow with ease.* Slowly and gently raise and lower your *right* eyebrow several times.

3. *Raise your eyelid with ease.* Slowly and gently raise and lower your right eyelid several times.

4. *Raise your eyes with ease.* With your eyes closed, slowly, gently allow your right eyeball to float upward, as if you were looking up, just above the horizon. Then, as you exhale, relax your eye.

5. *Put it all together.* Combine the movements of the eyebrow, eyelid, and eye into a single, effortless gesture.

Calming Mini-Move #4: Main Squeeze

1. *Secret handshake 1.* Place your hands in your lap with the palms facing down.

2. *Secret handshake 2.* Move your hands together and hold one of your thumbs.

3. *Secret handshake 3.* Extend the index finger of the grasping hand.

4. *Secret handshake 4.* Hold the extended index finger with the fingers of the other hand.

5. *Squeeze your thumb.* Slowly inhale, and as you do, gently, gradually squeeze your thumb. Then slowly exhale and gradually relax your grip on the thumb. Repeat several times, then rest for several complete breath cycles.

6. *Squeeze your index finger.* Slowly inhale, and as you do, gently, gradually squeeze your index finger. Then exhale, and as you do, gradually relax your grip on the finger. Repeat several times, then rest for several complete breath cycles or more.

7. *Alternate squeezes.* Slowly inhale, and as you do, gradually squeeze your thumb. Exhale, and gradually relax your grip. Then slowly inhale, and squeeze your index finger. Exhale, and relax your grip. Repeat several times, then rest for several complete breath cycles or more.

8. *Squeeze and look up.* Continue as before. But this time, each time you inhale and squeeze, allow your eyes to float upward. Your eyelids remain closed, but you raise your eyes as if you were looking up. Then exhale, relax your eyes, and relax your grip. Repeat several times, then rest for several complete breath cycles or more.

9. *To conclude.* Very gradually, as if by one molecule at a time, separate your hands and place them comfortably in your lap. Then very slowly open your eyes.

Calming Mini-Move #5: A Twist of the Wrists

1. *The Secret Handshake.* Join your hands in the Secret Handshake.

2. *A twist of the wrists.* Slowly inhale and, as you do, gently, gradually bend your wrists a little bit back, so your knuckles rise upward and the backs of your hand incline very slightly toward you. Exhale, and relax your wrists. Repeat several times, then rest for several complete breath cycles or more.

3. *Float your eyes up.* Slowly inhale, bend your wrists, and simultaneously allow your eyes to float upward. Then exhale, relax your eyes, and relax your wrists. Repeat several times, then rest for several complete breath cycles or more.

4. *Stop, rest, and feel.* Feel the result of the movements you have done.

Calming Mini-Move #6: Touching Your Heart

1. *Touch your heart.* Place the center of the palm of one of your hands over the center of your chest. Feel the warmth of your hand as it meets the warmth of your heart. Continue for several minutes or more. Then stop, rest, and feel.

2. *Touch your heart with both hands.* Place one hand over your heart, and the other hand on top of it. Make no effort. Breathe easy, and allow your hands to ride up and down with the gentle rising and falling of your breath. Continue for several minutes or more. Then stop, rest, and feel.

3. *Touch your heart with a smile.* Touch your heart with one or both hands, whichever you prefer. Allow your hands to ride up and down with the rising and falling of your breath. Each time you slowly inhale, *think a smile*. Each time you exhale, relax. Continue for several minutes or more. Then stop, rest, and feel.

Chapter 5
Lulling Mini-Move #1: Breath Surfing 1

1. *Home position.* The tips of the four fingers of both hands rest on either side of your chest. Your thumbs rest wherever it's most comfortable for you.

2. *Lift and lower your thumbs.* Slowly inhale, and as your chest rises, slowly and gradually raise your thumbs away from your chest a little tiny bit. Slowly exhale and relax your thumbs. Repeat several times, then rest for several complete breath cycles or more.

3. *Variation 1: Lighten your thumbs.* Slowly inhale, and as your chest rises, carrying the thumbs upward, you activate the muscles of your thumbs a tiny little bit, as if to make the thumbs a little lighter. You are lifting your thumbs without really lifting them. You're just *lightening* them. Then slowly exhale, and relax. Repeat several times, then rest for several complete breath cycles or more.

4. *Variation 2: Lift your thumbs in your imagination only.* Slowly inhale, and lift your thumbs in your imagination only. Slowly exhale, and relax.

5. *Variation 3.* Try Breath Surfing with your index, middle, ring, or little fingers instead of your thumbs.

6. *Variation 4.* Try Breath Surfing with your hands on the middle or lower breathing spaces, as described in L.E.S.S. Is More.

Lulling Mini-Move #2: Breath Surfing 2

1. *Home position.* Bring your fingertips to your sternum, or breastbone, just as you did in Breath Surfing 1.

2. *Go deeper. Step 1.* With the first breath, slowly inhale, and gradually lift your *right* thumb. Slowly exhale, and gradually lower your thumb.

3. *Go deeper. Step 2.* With your second breath, slowly inhale, and do nothing with your thumbs. Simply attend to your breath. Your chest rises and falls, and your thumbs rise and fall with it.

4. *Go deeper. Step 3.* With your third breath, slowly inhale, and gradually lift your *left* thumb. Slowly exhale, and gradually lower your thumb. Allow your breath to subside completely.

5. *Go deeper. Conclusion.* Rest quietly for *three* complete breath cycles or more. While you rest, continue to attend to the gentle rising and falling movements of your chest and your thumbs.

6. *Continue.* Repeat the entire sequence as desired, resting a little longer after each round.

Lulling Mini-Move #3: Rocking the Cradle

1. *Home position.* Lie on your back with your knees bent and your feet standing flat on the floor.

2. *Push away.* Slowly inhale, and as you do so, *think* of extending your legs. Apply gentle traction to the floor, as if you were pushing *away* from you. Slowly exhale, and relax. Your hips rock back: Your tailbone rises toward the ceiling and your waist sinks into the floor. Repeat several times, then straighten your legs and rest for several complete breath cycles, or more.

3. *Draw your feet toward you.* Bend your knees again. Slowly inhale, and *think* of drawing your feet a little bit *toward* you. Apply gentle traction to the floor, as if you were drawing your feet toward you. Your hips rock forward: Your waist lifts away from the floor and your tailbone sinks down. Slowly exhale, relax. Repeat several times, then straighten your legs and rest for several complete breath cycles, or more.

4. *Rock to and fro 1.* Bend your knees again. On the first breath, slowly inhale, and think of pushing your feet away. Your hips rock back. Slowly exhale, relax.

5. *Rock to and fro 2.* On the second breath, slowly inhale, and think of drawing your feet toward you. Your hips rock forward. Slowly exhale, relax. Repeat several times.

Lulling Mini-Move #4: Tongue in Cheek

1. *Tongue in cheek, home position.* Gently place the tip of your tongue at the inside of your right cheek, just to the right of the corner of your mouth. Slowly inhale and press the tongue outward against the tissues of the cheek.

2. *Other positions for the tongue.*

Lulling Mini-Move #5: The Ziggurat

1. *Stage 1.* Lie on your right side with your hips and knees bent. Slowly inhale, and as you do, tip your left hip down a tiny bit. Keep your hip where it is, and slowly exhale.

2. *Stage 2.* With your next breath, slowly inhale and as you do, move your left hip down a little bit farther. Keep your hip where it is, and slowly exhale.

3. *Stage 3.* With your third breath, slowly inhale and move your left hip still farther down. Keep your hip where it is, and slowly exhale.

4. *Stage 4.* Slowly inhale, keeping your hip where it is. Then, slowly exhale and *very gradually* allow your right hip to relax and return to its natural resting position.

5. *Stop, rest, and feel.* After you have done this four-stage movement *just once,* stop, rest, and feel for *three or more* complete breath cycles. Repeat as desired, resting after each round.

Lulling Mini-Move #6: Welcoming Sleep with Open Arms (Instead of Pacing the Floor)

1. *Home position.* Stand with feet parallel, your arms resting comfortably at your sides.

2. *Roll your arms outward.* Slowly inhale and as you do so gradually rotate your arms outward so the palms of your hands face forward.

3. *Roll your arms inward.* Slowly inhale and roll your arms *inward,* so the palms of your hands face *behind* you.

4. *Spread the thumb and index finger.* Slowly inhale and as you do so, very gently spread the thumb and the index finger of each hand apart from each other. Slowly exhale, relax your hands.

5. *Spread the thumb and the little finger.* Slowly inhale, and as you do, very gently spread your thumbs apart from your little fingers and your little fingers apart from your thumbs. Then slowly exhale, and relax your hands.

6. *Welcome sleep with open arms 1.* Slowly inhale, and as you do, turn your arms outward so your palms face forward. At

the same time, spread your thumbs apart from your index fingers. Slowly exhale, and relax.

7. *Welcome sleep with open arms 2.* Then slowly inhale, turn your arms inward so your palms face back, and spread your thumbs apart from your little fingers. Then slowly exhale, relax your arms, and relax your hands.

About the Author

* * * *

Michael Krugman is the founder of the Sounder Sleep System. He has been a Guild Certified Feldenkrais Teacher since 1987 and is a lifelong student of traditional methods of self-healing.

Mr. Krugman teaches and lectures widely on sleep, alertness, self-healing, and corporate wellness issues. He operates professional enhancement programs for health-care professionals all over the United States and in Europe. He has taught employees at Saatchi & Saatchi, HBO, and Equitable Insurance; patients at Cedars-Sinai and Torrance Memorial Medical Centers in Los Angeles; and patrol officers for the NYPD.

He has been featured in *Fortune* magazine, the *Village Voice, Sleep & Health, Yoga Chicago, Sport Life* (Spain), and other publications. A longtime resident of New York City, he currently resides in New Mexico.